COMMON SPICE OR WONDER DRUG?

GINGER
Health Care Rediscovers Its Roots

Paul Schulick

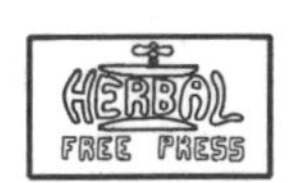

Herbal Free Press
Brattleboro, Vermont

Acknowledgments:
Special thanks to Mary Lou Quinn and Dr. Norman Farnsworth and all those who have worked on the Napralert project, the world's most complete database on natural remedies. Thanks also to my wife Barbi Schulick and my assistant Frances Harte for their invaluable editing and to all those who work on the shared vision to restore natural remedies to their rightful place.

Printed in the United States of America.

ISBN: 0-9639297-0-4

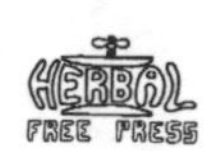

Herbal Free Press, Ltd.
RR1, Box 519
Brattleboro , VT 05301

Author's Note:

As remarkable and promising as the research on ginger is, it is important for the reader to recognize that there is no herb which can replace the value of exercise, good diet, healthy environment or a contented state of mind.

It is also critical that the reader understand that ginger cannot replace the expertise of a highly trained holistic health practitioner. Readers should consult with their practitioner before adopting the therapeutic applications in this book.

The author and publishers disclaim any liability arising directly or indirectly from the use of this book.

Table of Contents

Table of Figures

How to Use "Common Spice or Wonder Drug?"

This book is written with the hope of awakening an appreciation for ginger in lay persons and health professionals alike. Therefore, a format has been created that will facilitate the needs of those interested in gaining a quick general overview of ginger's healing potential as well as the scientific minded who desire a thorough understanding of ginger and its constituents.

- The more technical sections of the book have been prefaced with short comprehensive summaries called ☙ROOT NOTES❧ which may be the only reading of these sections needed for some.
- Less technical sections do not include ☙ROOT NOTES❧ and should prove informative for all readers.
- "The Essence of Ginger" on page 73 offers a succinct outline of main points.
- The Glossary on page 78 will aid in understanding unfamiliar terms.

It is hoped that the conclusions of *Common Spice or Wonder Drug?* will stimulate further research on this phenomenal, health-giving herb.

1

Beyond Sisyphus

In Greek mythology, Sisyphus, a king of Corinth, was condemned forever to roll a huge stone up a hill in Hades only to have it roll down again on nearing the top.

Your spice cabinet contains an herb possessing so many therapeutic applications that no modern drug can rival it. The plant, Zingiber officinale, commonly known as ginger, is one of the world's ten favorite spices,[1,2] yet astonishingly only a small fraction of its value is generally recognized.

Is it possible that a common spice can save tens of thousands of lives or billions of dollars in lost work days? If a lowly carrot (beta carotene) or a common citrus mold (penicillin) can offer substances which prevent disease or save millions of lives, why not a spice?

Unfortunately, over the past 40 years, the prevailing health-care system and the government agencies entrusted to regulate it have virtually excluded this possibility, along with many others related to so-called "alternative" or "traditional" medicine. Especially kept in competitive check have been the potential substitutions for modern pharmaceutical drugs which encompass herbs like ginger and other nutritional supplements. Physicians and various health-care providers who have recommended these supplements have suffered the indignity of being labeled "quacks," and more importantly have endured the threat of financially devastating licensor losses. In addition and not surprisingly, as of this writing, the supplements themselves–the "tools of the trade"–can be seized through the use of any number of absurd technicalities. For example, the government requires that anytime a health claim about an herb or dietary supplement is made, the producers must prove that this supplement is a safe and effective drug.

This "proving" sounds fair enough, but like Sisyphus and the rock it is a feat that is impossible to accomplish. A new drug application costs up to $359 million,[2a] takes eight or more years to process and most ironically can never actually result in a patent because an herb in its natural state is not a patentable substance. An herb, in other words, can never truly be a "drug" or be used for therapeutic reasons, according to the government's definition. Ultimately, as designed, only the pharmaceutical industry can create a therapeutic substance and sell to its sanctioned medical trade.

Despite this monopolistic pressure, growing numbers of Americans are seeking out alternative forms of health care. A recent survey in the most prestigious *New England Journal of Medicine* declared that in 1990 more than one-third of all Americans had visited an alternative practitioner. Perhaps more telling was the fact that "72 percent of the respondents who used unconventional therapy did not inform their medical doctor that they had done so."[2b]

It is most encouraging that this segment of the population has begun to organize into a politically active group. By forming grass-roots organizations throughout the United States, alternative health as a choice can now challenge the very roots of the health-care establishment and lift the historic and rightful representation of herbs and natural health care into the critical national debate on health-care reform. Through this consumer pressure, it is now possible that in the near future herbs may bc granted the therapeutic status and classification they well deserve, freeing them from the yoke of unattainable drug status requirements. Hopefully research like this on ginger will contribute to this all-important battle for healthier choices and medical freedom.

"Unless we put medical freedom into the Constitution, the time will come when medicine will organize itself into an undercover dictatorship. To restrict the art of healing to doctors and deny equal privileges to others will constitute the Bastille of medical science. All such laws are un-American and despotic."

Dr. Benjamin Rush,
Signer of the Declaration of Independence[3]

2

The Roots of Ginger

"Every good quality is contained in ginger."
An ancient Indian proverb

Botany 101

Ginger is one of hundreds of species belonging to the Zingiberaceae family sharing the family's most popular honors with the spice turmeric. It is a slender perennial reaching 24 to 39 inches in height. Its first stems are longer than the second and latter stems and bear flowers which are greenish-yellow and streaked with purple. The leaves are a dark green with a prominent midrib that is sheathed at the base and the seeds are found in the rare fruiting body.

The part that is used in commerce is the irregular-shaped and sized underground section commonly called a root and technically known as a rhizome. It is aromatic, thick-lobed and pale yellow in color.[4]

Ginger appears in many cultivated varieties, with an estimated fifty in India alone. Each variety possesses its own distinctive taste and aroma depending upon the soil and the manner in which it is grown.[5] Ginger grows best in a hot and moist climate with available shade, and in soil that is rich in loam and well tilled. When sold as fresh, ginger is harvested 5 to 6 months after planting, approximately three months earlier than the ginger processed for dried powders.[6]

Approximately 8 pounds of fresh rhizome are necessary to produce 1 pound of dried herb.

An Illustrious Past

> "Ginger is perhaps the best and most sattvic [life-supporting] of the spices. It was called *vishwabhesaj*, the universal medicine."
>
> *Dr. Vasant Lad*[7]

Ginger originated in the tropics of Southeast Asia. There was a time when ginger was actually worshipped as a healing gift from God. In ancient India, ginger was

Figure 1

The History of Ginger's Worldwide Movement[10]

Native to Southeast Asia and widely used since the earliest written records in India and China.

3000 B.C.	Described in Greek Literature[11]
551-479 B.C.	Described by Confucius
1st century	Described by Romans Pliny andDioscorides
176 A.D.	Taxed in Alexandria, Egypt
9th century	Appeared Widely Throughout Europe
1280-1290	Harvest Described by Marco Polo
1292	Harvest Described by Italian Montecorvine
13th century	Introduced by Arabs into East Africa
1416	Introduced into Malacca, Malaysia
1547	Intoduced into West Indies by Spaniard de Mendoza
16th century	Intoduced by Portuguese into West Africa; Recommended by Henry VIII as Plague Cure
19th century	Ginger Beer Consumed as Popular English Tavern Drink
1920	Introduced into Australia

given the name *vishwabhesaj* or "the universal medicine."[8] This reverence is still demonstrated today in the Orient where ginger remains a component of more than fifty percent of all traditional herbal remedies.[7,9]

Ginger is cited in the classic literature of Buddhist, Arabic, Greek and Roman cultures and in the records of explorers Marco Polo and Vasco da Gama.[11] Reports differ as to the first references to ginger, one dates back to Greece five thousand years ago.[12] *(See Figure 1.)*

Appreciation for ginger's medicinal properties was superseded in the Middle Ages by the political power it represented. Ginger helped shape nations and change the course of modern history as the wealth and power of historic empires were measured in part by their trade in spices. Ginger was one of the key spices which sent Europeans around the globe. Wars were fought and new worlds discovered in the race to gain access to the spice trade routes. The Spaniards were particularly aggressive explorers, taking the plant from India and Southeast Asia to the West Indies and Mexico. In medieval Europe the culinary experience of ginger was one reserved only for royalty.

"It is of an heating and digesting qualitie, and is profitable for the stomacke."

John Gerard, 1597[13]

It can be argued that herbal medicine's use of ginger reached its peak in the United States in the early 20th century with references in multiple editions of Ellingwood's great tome *Materia Medica Therapeutics and Pharmacognosy.* Finley Ellingwood, M.D., relied upon the observations of approximately 25,000 physicians, called eclectics, to bring this work to completion.

The following quotes from the eclectics suggest their profound appreciation for ginger. While emphasis is placed on the digestive properties, some of ginger's sustained effects as an anti-inflammatory, systemic regulator and circulatory tonic were clearly noted.

"When chewed it occasions an increased flow of saliva, and when swallowed it acts as a stimulating tonic, stomachic, and carminative, increasing the secretion of gastric juice, exalting the excitability of the alimentary muscular system, and dispelling gases accumulated in the stomach and bowels....It is eminently useful in habitual flatulency, atonic dyspepsia, hysteria and enfeebled and relaxed habits, especially of old and gouty individuals; and is excellent to relieve nausea, pains and cramps of the stomach and bowels...especially when those conditions are due to colds....Ginger in the form of 'ginger tea' is popular and efficient as a remedy for breaking up colds, and in relieving the pangs of disordered menstruation."

Harvey Wickes Felter, M.D., and John Uri Lloyd, Phr.M., Ph.D.[14]

"The hot decoction of ginger tea is an excellent diaphoretic for breaking up incipient colds. It stimulates the circulation and the warmth it imparts to the body corrects the surface chilliness associated with colds....It stimulates the flow of the digestive juices and the warmth it imparts to the stomach is gratifying."

A. W. Kuts-Cheraux, N.D.[15]

"It is a profound and immediate stimulant, an active diaphoretic, an anodyne in gastric and intestinal pain, and a sedative to an irritated and overwrought system when there is extreme exhaustion."

Finley Ellingwood, M.D., and John Uri Lloyd, Ph.M., Ph.D., LL.D.[16]

Although many of the historic claims for ginger are not yet backed by double-blind placebo-controlled studies (a condition which will hopefully change in the near future), this should not diminish the profound value of historic observation.

If a remedy is used for hundreds or even thousands of years for a particular purpose, it is highly doubtful that its popularity could be sustained if it were a placebo effect alone. Why would parents throughout history give their feverish children ginger if it didn't work?

From the Admiralty Islands to Yemen, the list of traditionally tested treatments using ginger is monumental. *(See Figure 2.)*

More significantly, if a therapeutic application is used for the same purpose in completely different regions of the world, this clearly suggests there is authenticity to the usage. As an example, it is beyond coincidence that ginger has been used as a treatment for arthritis from Brazil to the Sudan to Papua-New Guinea, as an emmenagogue (to promote menstruation) from Venezuela to Vietnam, and as an aphrodisiac from Cuba to Yemen.

Lastly, it is undeniable that common sense plays a crucial part in the scientific method. Although there are beginning to be well-designed studies supporting or confirming many of the historic claims for ginger, some of these claims are virtually irrefutable. Just as studies are unnecessary to confirm the stimulant action of coffee or the laxative effect of prunes, ginger's value as a digestive tonic is unequivocal.

Figure 2
Historic Values of Ginger *□

Admiralty Islands:
- contraceptive[17]

Brazil:
- bronchitis[18]
- rheumatism

China:
- emmenagogue[19]
- digestive tonic[20]
- metabolic increase[21]

Cuba:
- emmenagogue[22]
- systemic stimulant
- aphrodisiac

England:
- morning sickness[23]

Fiji:
- coughs[24]
- colds
- stomach ache
- asthma
- ear ache

India:
- emmenagogue[25]
- dietary vegetable[26]
- ulcerative gingivitis[27]
- filariasis[28]
- ease delivery[29]
- tuberculosis
- sore throat
- stomach pain[30]
- headache
- digestive stimulant
- colic
- carminative
- cough[20]
- fever
- rheumatism
- diabetes[31]
- nerve disorders[32]

Japan:
- hair growth[33]

Indonesia:
- colic[34]
- snakebite poultice
- rheumatic poultice

Malaysia:
- tonic after birth[35]

Mauritius:
- emmenagogue[36]

Mexico:
- digestive tonic[37]

Nigeria:
- schistosomiasis[38]
- wound healing[39]
- antimicrobial

Papua-New Guinea:
- migraine[40]
- vomiting
- poisonous stings
- digestive tonic
- colds[41]
- cough
- stomach worms
- toothache[41,42]
- malaria[42]
- aching limbs
- pneumonia
- tuberculosis
- fever
- rheumatism
- topical ulcers
- stomach problems[42]

Peru:
- carminative[43]
- contraceptive[44]

Philippines:
- childbirth pain[45]

Saudi Arabia:
- digestive[46-47]
- diuretic
- antiseptic
- carminative
- anesthetic
- astringent
- anti-emetic[20,47]
- carminative[20]

South Korea:
- abortifacient[48]

Sudan:
- colds, pneumonia[49]
- rheumatism

Sumatra:
- childbirth[35]

Tanganyika:
- galactagogue[50-51]

Thailand:
- tonic[52]
- anti-emetic[53]
- anticolic
- carminative[52-53]
- hypnotic
- cardiotonic
- postnatal[54]
- emmenagogue[54,56]
- digestive[55]
- fever[56]
- diarrhea
- carminative[57]
- headache

USA:
- carminative[58]
- digestive pain[14]
- antinausea
- cold remedy[15]
- diaphoretic
- antipyretic
- emmenagogue[16]
- migraines
- alcoholic gastritis[59]

Venezuela:
- emmenagogue[60]

Vietnam:
- emmenagogue[61]

Yemen:
- aphrodisiac[62]
- stimulant

** This table does not include references to ginger in multi-component formulas.*
□ First reference covers following values until the next citation.

The above chart documents how ginger has been used around the world. Many of these applications can now be justified through modern research.

3

Eicosanoids & Other Light Subjects

As fascinating and diverse as ginger's historical applications are, the past thirty years of scientific investigation offer a significantly broader panorama of untapped health potential. This chapter offers insight into the mechanisms of how ginger actually prevents or benefits conditions like life-threatening heart attacks, arthritis and ulcers. A fringe benefit in both Chapters 3 and 4 are parcels of information which address important questions in the larger puzzle of modern health science, such as:

- How valid or safe is the quest in modern drug development for a botanical's "active principle?"
- How do herbs compare in effectiveness and safety with modern drugs?
- How significant is the potential toxicity of a single compound in a plant?
- What is the rationale behind the ancient assertion that there is a synergy and art to herbal combination?

Eicosanoids & Other Light Subjects

This chapter contains complex topics dealing with questions to which whole books or journals are devoted. While this chapter is at risk of being rudimentary to the professional and potentially slow reading to the layperson, it is important to an appreciation of how ginger works and its profound healing potential.

An Infinite Cascade of Reactions

ROOT NOTES

One of the most challenging questions facing a student of herbal medicine today is to explain how an herb works or brings about a desired effect. Underlying one simple observed effect like ginger's relief of inflammation might be a dozen different complex chemical or principal interactions. Although ginger's actions are possibly beyond comprehension, understanding something about these mechanisms or simply that they exist might help the student better appreciate, use and gain value from the herb.

Ginger's observed effects are the result of an almost infinite cascade of reactions caused by literally hundreds of individual compounds. Research into these compounds began to be carefully investigated in the 1880's with the extraction of an oily-resinous substance, composing approximately five to ten percent of the plant.[63] This oleoresin was further broken down into two of ginger's distinctive active elements called gingerols and shogaols.

Although gingerols and shogaols are still considered today to be the principal active group of constituents, more than 300 additional compounds have now been studied and classified.[64] Many of these elements are "active," meaning if isolated, they will possess a distinctive physiological effect. For example, the active principles gingerenone A and [6]-gingerol are recognized as antifungal agents and antiemetics respectively.[65] *(See Figure 3.)*

Figure 3
The Complexity of Effect

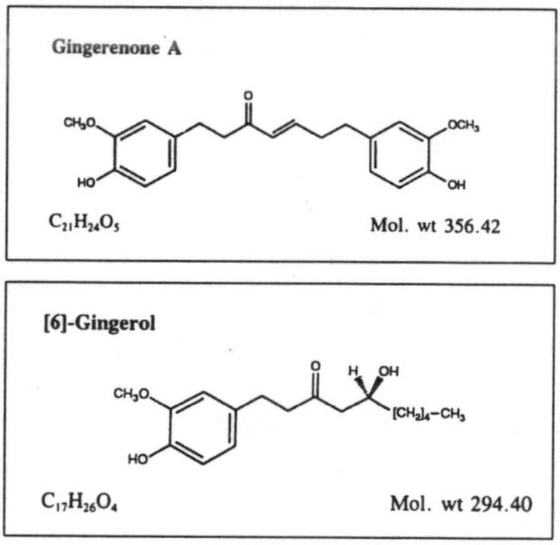

Gingerenone A

$C_{21}H_{24}O_5$ Mol. wt 356.42

[6]-Gingerol

$C_{17}H_{26}O_4$ Mol. wt 294.40

Chemical structures have been described for literally hundreds of the constituents of ginger. The above structures are included as examples of two with defined physiological activities.[66]

When these active constituents are combined with other active or "inactive" compounds, those activities are intensified, modified or negated and collectively become what are referred to here as "principal actions."◆ Principal actions either alone or more typically in combination result in a myriad of "observed effects." Without trying to make it too complicated, an observed effect can also have at its roots a variety of principal actions. *(See Figure*

◆ Further examples of the interplay of plant constituents are detailed in the sections, "Ulcers–The $2.8 Billion Challenge" (pg. 29) and "Getting at the Roots of Cancer" (pg. 46). See "Ginger's Constituents & Actions" (pg. 85) for a chart of ginger's more than 300 elements and their known properties.

Figure 4
The Interplay of Actions & Effects

Singular Action Can Create Multiple Observed Effects

Principal Action	**Observed Effects**
Enzyme	Improved Digestion, Antibacterial, Anthelmintic, Anti-inflammatory

Singular Observed Effect Can Result From Multiple Principal Actions

Observed Effect	**Principal Actions**
Anti-inflammatory	Enzyme, Eicosanoid Balance, Antioxidant

4.) Understanding the basics of these cause and effect relationships will allow the reader to more fully appreciate the profound therapeutic benefits of ginger.

Ginger's principal enzyme action[67-69] is a good example of one with numerous observed effects. One of the enzymes which participates in ginger's enzyme action is called zingibain and it is more potent than either papain from papaya or ficin from figs, comprising about two percent of the fresh juice.[67-68] One gram of zingibain can actually tenderize as much as 20 pounds of meat.[69] Improved digestion is the clearest impact or observed effect of ginger's enzyme action.

Ginger's principal enzyme action also undoubtedly contributes to its antibacterial[70-72] and anthelmintic observed effects.[39,73-81] Numerous studies have shown that enzymes like zingibain can enhance the effectiveness of other antibacterial elements such as antibiotics[82-87] by as much as 50 percent.[83] To help eliminate parasites, an enzyme like zingibain can also aid the immune system by potentially digesting the parasite and its eggs.[88]

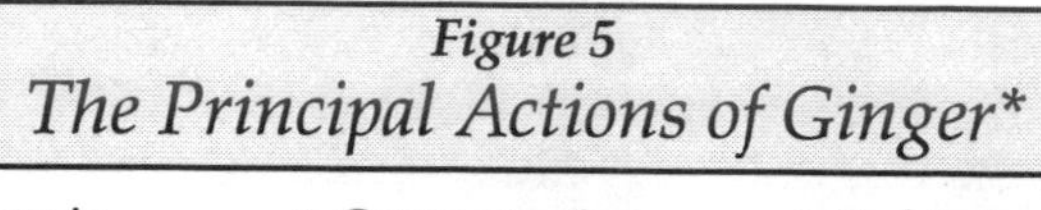

Figure 5
*The Principal Actions of Ginger**

○ Adaptogenic	○ Cytoprotection	○ Probiotic
○ Antioxidant	○ Eicosanoid Balance	○ Serotonin Balance
○ Antitoxic	○ Enzyme	○ Stimulant
○ Bioavailability		

*See glossary for definitions

Ginger's potent anti-inflammatory properties[20,32,72,89-96] exemplify an observed effect with at least three principal actions at its root: (1) enzyme, (2) eicosanoid balance and (3) antioxidant.

Through a complex synergistic effect, principal enzyme action combines with at least four other ginger constituents to modulate another principal action involving inflammation-related elements which are called eicosanoids.[20,97-101]

Figure 6
*Ginger's Demonstrated Effects**

Analgesic	Anti-bacterial	Anti-cathartic
Anti-diabetic	Anti-emetic	Anti-fungal
Anthelmintic	Anti-inflammatory	Anti-mutagenic
Anti-thrombic	Antitussive	Anti-ulcer
Anti-viral	Anti-tumor	Hypocholesteremic
Immune Supportive	Thermoregulatory	

*See glossary for definitions

Lastly, ginger's principal antioxidant◆ action[102-110] is also related to its observed anti-inflammatory effect. Without doubt, the relationship between inflammation and inhibition of free radicals is widely accepted. Ginger is rated in a number of studies to possess a free radical-inhibiting index even greater than that of commercial antioxidant preservatives BHA and BHT.[103-105]

What is the interplay between ginger's digestive enzymes and antioxidants? Which element is most responsible for the observed anti-inflammatory effect? Those are questions even the most elaborate research may never answer.

Connecting a plant's active elements with clinically observed effects is probably a valuable exercise but a Herculean task and not attempted here. With this in mind, please note on page 14: Figure 5, "The Principal Actions of Ginger" and Figure 6, "Ginger's Demonstrated Effects."

◆ Ginger's antioxidant action is thought to result from a number of constituents including zingerone.

The Fleckless Balance

☙ ROOT NOTES ❧

One of the body's most important chemical reactions involves compounds called eicosanoids (pronounced 'ikosanoydz'). When these elements, which are derived from dietary fat, are out of balance, many different disease conditions can evolve. Two of the most threatening problems which can result from this imbalance are heightened inflammation and a more viscous or clot-prone blood. To a person who is susceptible to arthritis or heart disease, the results of this imbalance could be devastating. Drug companies have spent many billions of dollars unsuccessfully attempting to manipulate this balance.

There is little doubt that another key to understanding the benefits of ginger is to appreciate its relationship with compounds called eicosanoids. Since this single connection is so critical to the observed effects of ginger, all later sections in this book inevitably touch upon it.

Eicosanoids are those physiologically active compounds, enzymatically produced from fatty acids and possessing a hormonal or regulatory-type nature. Eicosanoids are broken down into three major groups depending upon their structure. *(See Figure 7.)*

Prostaglandins (PG), first isolated from the prostate gland in the 1930's and now identifiable in virtually all other body tissues, constitute a minimum of thirty different compounds with innumerable physiological effects.

Thromboxanes (TX) are produced mainly by blood

platelets and among other effects are responsible for platelet aggregation or clotting.

Leukotrienes (LT), first isolated from white blood cells, mediate inflammatory or allergic responses.

All three groups interact with each other in virtually every organ system of the body. For example in the mesangial cells of the kidney, specific prostaglandins and thromboxanes named (TX)A2 and (PG)E2alpha perform a contractile effect, while others, PGE2 and PGI2, are relaxant.[111]

Eicosanoids are in a state of constant flux and must maintain a balance for health to be preserved. As tempting as it is to classify one eicosanoid as "bad" and another as "good," the reality is that each is vital and its ratio or proportion with the others is probably the most important factor. Even the leukotrienes, which are usually blamed for chronic inflammatory conditions such as asthma, rheumatoid arthritis, psoriasis and inflammatory bowel disease,[112-114] clearly play a role in the destruction

Figure 7

The Three Eicosanoids & Their Enzymes

Eicosanoids	**Enzymes**
Prostaglandins (PG)	Cyclooxygenase
Thromboxanes (TX)	Cyclooxygenase, Thromboxane synthetase
Leukotrienes (LT)	5-Lipoxygenase

Other enzymes involved in eicosanoid synthesis are: E2 isomerase, I2 synthase, 12-lipoxygenase and cytochrome P-450.

Eicosanoid production depends upon numerous enzymes. Drug companies have encountered serious side effects when attempting to modulate these enzymes.

of harmful materials and contribute to tissue repair and healing.

A good example of the eicosanoid dynamic occurs during pregnancy. All reproductive tissues can create certain prostaglandins and thromboxanes. PGI2 (also called prostacyclin) and TXA2 production are important regulators of the fetal blood supply. PGI2 dilates and makes the blood less sticky while TXA2 constricts and causes blood aggregation.

Figure 8
The Thromboxane–Prostacyclin Balance

Thromboxane Enzyme Modulation

Thromboxane synthetase (TS) excess

Excess cellular calcium	Excess inflammatory 2 series	Impaired renal function
Unexplained infertility	Arteriosclerosis	Coronary artery spasm
Sudden death	Cardiac arrhythmias	Pulmonary hypertension
Anxiety	Psoriasis	Depression
Muscular dystrophy		

Thromboxane synthetase (TS) inhibition

Counters adult respiratory distress syndrome	Enhances vitamin E
Reduces platelet deposition	Prevents peptic ulceration
Reduces myocardial injury impact	Counters traumatic shock

Prostacyclin (PGI2) Dominance*

Counters peripheral arterial disease	Counteracts TXA2
Anti-aggregatory	Blocks arrhythmias
Stabilizes lysosomal membranes	Counters ischemic strokes
Regulates allergic/inflammation	Modulates immune reactions
Lowers blood pressure	Antimetastatic agent

Figure 8 summarizes the work of researcher Joshua Backon detailing some of the implications of fluctuations in just one enzyme and eicosanoid.[120] The impact of these two interrelated systems is remarkable. From the data it is safe to conclude that a moderated level of thromboxanes and a prostacyclin dominance is systemically desirable. Research demonstrates that ginger inhibits (TS) while maintaining (PGI2) dominance.

In a normal pregnancy, PGI2, which is widely accepted as being a most important prostaglandin, dominates over TXA2. During complications with pregnancy like pre-eclampsia and multiple abortions, PGI2 decreases and TXA2 increases. Interestingly, smoking, associated with increased birth defects, also decreases the ratio of the eicosanoid PGI2 to TXA2.[115]

Obviously, eicosanoid manipulation is the key to the normal functioning of many body systems (i.e., the inflammatory process and cardiovascular system). Because of this, modern drug companies have attempted to modulate eicosanoid enzymes like thromboxane synthetase and cyclooxygenase. *(See Figure 8 on previous page.)* To date, at least 200 drugs[89] have been specifically designed to manipulate eicosanoids or relieve the inflammatory process at a current marketing and development cost as high as *$70 billion.*

Unfortunately the drug companies have encountered serious problems when trying to manipulate either the thromboxane synthetase or cyclooxygenase enzymes.[89-90,116-127]

When thromboxane synthetase is inhibited, other prostaglandin-type substances called prostaglandin endoperoxides replace the thromboxanes. The unfortunate result is the forces of contraction and aggregation still dominate.[118] To make matters worse, thromboxane synthetase inhibitors are also known to hamper normal removal of calcium from cells and lead to overproduction of other inflammatory prostaglandins like PGF2 alpha.[120]

When the cyclooxygenase enzyme pathway is checked with non-steroidal anti-inflammatory drugs (NSAIDs), like aspirin, ibuprofen and indomethacin, the prostaglandin balance is likewise upset. NSAIDs reduce prostaglandins like PGI2 leading to a breakdown in the protective linings of the stomach and kidneys and consequently resulting in potentially fatal ulcers.[116,121-126,173]

The greatest concern of chemical eicosanoid manipulation however is probably not ulcers, "rebound" inflammation or hypertension,[127] rather it could be a significant compromise of the immune system. Eicosanoids play a key role in immune function and their inhibition could dramatically affect immunity.[128-133]

A Key to the $70 Billion Vault

ROOT NOTES

Remarkably, ginger, a mere inexpensive spice, proves superior to multi-billion dollar pharmaceuticals in correcting an all-important enzyme balance that is a key to quality of life and longevity.

The most remarkable and probably important principal action of ginger is that it is a profound and safe modulator or balancer of the vital eicosanoid cascade.

In numerous studies ginger and at least four of its individual compounds have been shown to correct eicosanoid ratios (inhibiting excesses of thromboxanes and leukotrienes such as TXA2 and LTB4) while vital prostaglandins like PGI2 remain dominant.[20,32,72,89-91,93-96,101,120] Estimates range from a 37 percent inhibition of thromboxanes to a 56 percent inhibition in specific inflammatory-type prostaglandins.[72,93-94] *(See Figure 9.)*

Ginger achieved this inhibition without any compromise to the immune phagocytosis response.[72] And, unlike any comparable drug, ginger also reduced the "substitute" inflammatory compounds called prostaglandin endoperoxides.[94]

The impact of the eicosanoid-balancing action of ginger is truly far reaching and probably impossible to completely quantify. Just as a wholesome meal can nourish and uplift every system of the body, balancing of eicosanoids will bring profound systemic benefits.

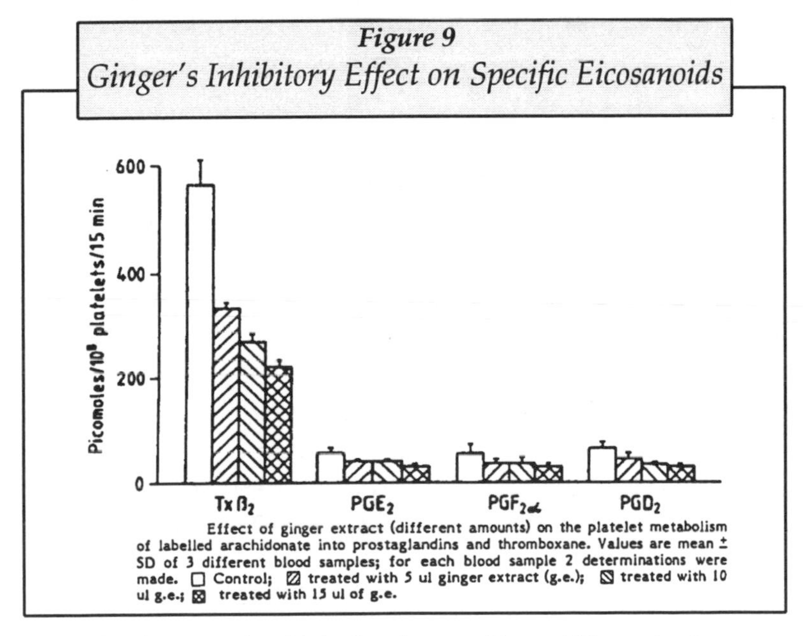

The above graph published in the noted journal "Prostaglandins, Leukotrienes and Medicine" illustrates how ginger significantly inhibits certain thromboxanes (TX) and prostaglandins (PG) which can contribute to inflammation and thrombosis.[134]

4

Ginger: The Healer

Chapter 4 details the fantastic range of therapeutic values for one of nature's safest, easiest and most enjoyable herbs to consume. It will become clear that this readily available spice is capable of improving a wide variety of human infirmities from arthritis to ulcers while it tones or strengthens virtually every organ system of the body.

Relief for 27 Million Painful Days

ROOT NOTES

Modern medicine has had little to offer in treating arthritis, the nation's primary crippler. Side effects plague these conventional medications killing thousands each year and it is a rare event when the patient is actually healed. In two clinical trials conducted in Denmark, ginger actually reversed many of the subjects' arthritic symptoms and did so without side effects. Researchers attributed the benefit to the balancing of critical body enzymes.

"After the diagnosis of rheumatoid arthritis all patients were treated with non-steroidal anti-inflammatory drugs (NSAIDs) and some of the patients in later stages with corticosteroids and/or with gold salts. All the above management treatments only provided temporary relief...Patient 1, an Asian male of fifty years of age living in Canada was diagnosed as having rheumatoid arthritis. This patient began consumption of ginger in the first month following diagnosis by taking about fifty grams of fresh ginger daily after light cooking along with vegetables and various meats...Pain and inflammation subsided after 30 days of ginger consumption. After consuming fifty grams of ginger daily for three months the subject was completely free of pain, inflammation or swelling. He has continued to perform his job as automechanic without any relapses of arthritis for the last 10 years."

K.C. Srivastava[90]

The range of diseases that ginger can positively affect as an anti-inflammatory agent is staggering. Some of the conditions with chronic inflammation or eicosanoid imbalance at the root are asthma,[112,135-136] painful menstruation[137-138] and migraine.[137-142◆]

Probably the best example of ginger's anti-inflammatory potential is in the treatment of arthritis, "the nation's primary crippler."[89] Although more than 100 different diseases are grouped together under the designation arthritis,[143] the common thread among them is inflammation. It is estimated that 80 percent of persons over the age of 50 suffer from "osteoarthritis,"[144] while rheumatoid arthritis, a chronic inflammatory disease which affects the entire body including the joints, inflicts as many as 7 million in the United States.[145] Besides the incalculable cost of pain, arthritis is estimated

◆ A recently published case history of a migraine sufferer who experienced relief from ginger comparable to the drug dihydroergotamine underlined ginger's potential.[32]

to result in the loss of 27 million work days or $8.6 billion in the U.S. alone.[89]

In the past one hundred years, there has been little progress in the treatment of arthritis. This is made painfully clear in the writings of Sir William Osler, a 19th century British physician, and Wallace Epstein who is currently professor of medicine at the University of California, San Francisco.

"When a patient with arthritis walks in the front door, I feel like leaving out the back door."

Sir William Osler[89]

"No one really knows whether prednisone, gold injections, methotrexate, sulfasalazine or hydroxychloroquine alter the joint destruction and deformity associated with the disease (arthritis)... Physicians do so without solid evidence that they do more good than harm in the long run. Ten years after commencing treatment, virtually no rheumatoid arthritis patients still take these medications, either because they do not work, or because of side effects."

Wallace V. Epstein[146]

Two clinical trials in Denmark strongly suggest that ginger should be included in all arthritis treatment programs.[89-90]

In the first trial performed in 1989, 7 rheumatic patients consumed fresh or powdered ginger for a period of three months. All patients reported that ginger "produced better relief of pain, swelling and stiffness than the administration of NSAIDs." Remarkably six of these seven patients had been "continuously afflicted with some degree of pain, inflammation, swelling and morning stiffness even after five to ten years of diagnosis and conventional treatment."

In the second trial involving 56 patients (28 with rheumatoid arthritis, 18 with osteoarthritis and 10 with muscular discomfort), the author K.C. Srivastava concluded that "more than three-quarters experienced, to varying degrees, relief in pain and swelling. All the patients with muscular discomfort experienced relief in pain."

Although both Danish studies mostly attributed the benefits to balancing of eicosanoids, it can be argued that many other principal actions of ginger are at play.

An important note is that during the 2.5 year period of ginger consumption, no side effects were reported. Considering that conventional arthritis treatment annually results in 3,300 NSAIDs-induced ulcer deaths among the elderly alone,[147] ginger's advantage is clear.

"Ginger produced better relief of pain, swelling and stiffness than the administration of NSAIDs...Some of our (arthritis) patients have observed added benefits on taking ginger, and they include relief in cold sores...fewer colds, amelioration of stomach irritation and constipation."

K.C. Srivastava[89-90]

Common Spice or Wonder Drug?

Your Heart Wants Ginger, Not Aspirin

☙ ROOT NOTES ❧

Today's lifestyles wreak havoc on the circulatory system. In an attempt to correct the problem, modern medicine is now suggesting regular intake of aspirin to prevent life-threatening strokes and heart attacks. Although the prescription sounds strange, it does have an element of value behind it which many researchers say could save hundreds of thousands of lives. Their justification is: by inhibiting a specific enzyme, aspirin makes the blood less prone to dangerous clotting. The downside is that aspirin has a long precarious list of potential side effects. Amazingly, ginger not only inhibits this same enzyme but it does so without side effects.

More than one-half of all deaths occurring in the United States annually are caused by "clogged arteries." Included in the catastrophic results of clogged arteries are heart attacks, coronary and cerebral thromboses, very high blood pressure, angina pectoris, shock, strokes and heart failure.[148]

A major contributor to clogged arteries is an excess of platelet-generated thromboxanes. Excess thromboxanes increase blood viscosity and aggregation leading to lethal clotting. Many physicians now recommend the daily intake of acetylsalicylic acid (aspirin) to check this phenomenon and reduce the number of fatal heart attacks.

Because of aspirin's specific inhibitory effect on thromboxanes, it is estimated that regular consumption could prevent 600,000 heart attacks a year and 200,000 heart attack deaths. Research also suggests that regular consumption of the thromboxane-inhibitor could prevent 25,000 stroke-related deaths and as many as 24,000 deaths from colo-rectal cancer.[149] However, it is well known that aspirin, like other NSAIDs, possesses significant adverse side effects.

Ginger and at least one of its constituents clearly possess a similar ability to inhibit thromboxanes and platelet aggregation.[92-95,128,150] However, compared to aspirin, ginger is far safer and offers a host of other benefits. Compared to other natural products, such as garlic, that are recommended for their anti-aggregatory properties, ginger is clearly superior.[92-93,95] Considering that even the smallest amount of ginger extract can "abolish" aggregation[93] and that literally hundreds of thousands of lives can be saved emphasizes that ginger should be included in everyone's daily supplement routine.

One cannot leave the discussion of ginger as a therapeutic agent for the cardiovascular system without a brief mention of its principal antioxidant action.

> "The evidence is accumulating that people who are taking an antioxidant of some sort seem to have a high degree of protection from coronary heart disease."
>
> *Dr. Claude Lenfant*
>
> *Director of the National Heart, Lung and Blood Institute*[151]

As previously discussed, ginger is a powerful antioxidant, more so than even chemical antioxidants BHA and BHT. If, as noted researchers like Dr. Claude Lenfant suggest,[152] even a small amount of antioxidants can offer significant protection to the cardiovascular system, then there is yet another justification for ginger supplementation.

Whether the Heat Is High or Low

☙ ROOT NOTES ❧

Question. Why has ginger throughout time been a valuable aid in alleviating the fever and chills of colds? *Answer.* Ginger reduces fever for the same reason aspirin does. It inhibits the activity of a "fever causing" enzyme.

Ginger possesses profound thermoregulatory properties.[21,72,153-159] Like aspirin and other NSAIDs which inhibit certain inflammatory eicosanoids, ginger can alleviate the severity of a fever. When fever was induced in laboratory rats, ginger's effect was comparable to aspirin, reducing the fever by 38 percent.[72] Historical and modern research show that ginger is not simply limited to fever reduction but is also capable of relieving "chills caused by common cold and warming the body."[153-154]

Ulcers–The $2.8 Billion Challenge

☙ ROOT NOTES ❧

Ginger combines two effects beyond the scope of any modern drug. It can relieve inflammation while simultaneously protecting the digestive system from ulcers. A modern drug may accomplish one or the other but never both. Ginger possesses the valuable properties of modern antiulcer drugs but without the potential for negative side effects.

The Final Word on NSAIDs

"A medical knowledge that works–no matter how scientific its origins–is a treasure that cannot be ignored."

Dr. Hiroshi Nakajima,
Director General, World Health Organization.[89]

Whatever advantage NSAIDs have in the strength of their anti-inflammatory or thermoregulatory effects, ginger compensates for it with an absence of side effects and alternative benefits. One of these benefits is ginger's ulcer-preventive properties.[160-172] *(See Figure 10.)* At least six anti-ulcer constituents from ginger have been isolated and identified.[160-162]

Unlike NSAIDs which can cause life-threatening ulcers by inhibiting mucosal-protective prostaglandins, ginger maintains the vital eicosanoid balance and actually preserves the integrity of the digestive tract

Figure 10

Ginger's Ulcer–Protective Spectrum

Ginger Extract vs. Ulcer-Causing Agents

Procedure	Ulcer Index Control	Mean ± S.E. Ginger Ext (500 mg/kg P.O.)
80% Ethanol	7.62 ± 0.18	0.75 ± 0.25*
0.6% M HCL	7.12 ± 0.29	1.50 ± 1.89*
0.2 M NaOH	6.87 ± 0.29	1.12 ± 1.24*
25% NaCl	5.87 ± 0.35	1.37 ± 0.18*

**P< 0.001 Student's t-test as compared to respective controls.*
Eight animals were used in each group.

Ginger Extract vs. (NSAIDs)

Treatment	Dose mg/kg i.g.	Ulcer Index Mean ± S.E	P. value Student's t-test
Indomethacin			
Control	–	54.8 ± 7.40	–
Ginger	500	34.5 ± 2.3	< 0.05
Aspirin			
Control	–	33.0 ± 2.11	–
Ginger	500	19.6 ± 3.3	< 0.01

Eight animals were used in each group.

Researchers concluded from the above figures that ginger possesses a "significant cytoprotective" activity by increasing the resistance of the stomach protective mucus against noxious chemicals like hydrochloric acid and alcohol. Ginger also significantly reduced NSAIDs-induced ulcers. [164]

mucosa.[171-172] When laboratory animals are exposed to severe stress from either immobilization in water or chemical-induced lesions, whole ginger extract inhibits ulcers by as much as 97.5 percent.[162] (Notably, two of ginger's most "active" constituents, [6]-gingerol and zingiberene, only inhibited gastric lesions by 53 and 54 percent respectively, supporting the contention that the whole plant is superior to individual constituents.)

NSAIDs may relieve inflammation but their treatment course will inevitably lead to the need for new drugs, or what can be referred to as "domino drugs." Ironically one of ginger's advantages over NSAIDs is it that it can be significantly "cytoprotective" against even the ulcers that NSAIDs themselves actually induce.[164]

Protecting against NSAIDs-induced ulcers is no minor achievement as these ulcers are recognized as being "often unresponsive to H2-receptor antagonists."[173]

Ginger Takes on the H2s

For the 25 million American males and 12 million females who suffer from duodenal and gastric ulcers,[174] the daily consumption of ginger offers an attractive alternative to Zantac® (ranitidine), Pepcid® (famotidine) and Tagamet® (cimetidine).◆ These three drugs, which are collectively referred to as H2-receptor antagonists, are notably among the twenty top-selling drugs in the U.S., and account for approximately $2.8 billion in sales annually.[175] *(See Figure 11.)*

Ginger has distinct advantages over these H2-receptor antagonists.□ Besides its observed effect against NSAIDs-induced ulcers, ginger has two other benefits in its favor: (1) more optimal maintenance of pepsin-pH pa-

◆ Zantac® is a registered trademark of the Glaxo Inc., Pepcid® is a registered trademark of Merck & Co. and Tagamet® is a registered trademark of Smithkline Beecham.

□ The advantage of ginger over H2s as a protective agent against ulcers would probably be even greater with the simple addition of licorice. Numerous studies[176a-e] on licorice and its constituents show a profound healing property once lesions have formed.

Figure 11
The Twenty Top-Selling Drugs for 1992
(By U.S. Sales in Millions)

RANK	BRAND	PRODUCT TYPE	MARKETER	U.S. SALES
1	**ZANTAC**	Antiulcer agent	Glaxo Inc.	$1,734.60
2	Procardia line	Antihypertensive/antianginal	Pfizer Inc.	$1,100.00
3	Mevacor	Cholesterol reducer	Merck & Co., Inc.	$1,040.00
4	Cardizem line	Antihypertensive/antianginal	Marion Merrell Dow Inc.	$ 922.00
5	Vasotec	Antihypertensive	Merck & Co., Inc.	$ 835.00
6	Prozac	Antidepressant	Eli Lilly and Co.	$ 835.00
7	**TAGAMET**	Antiulcer agent	SmithKline Beecham	$ 647.50
8	Ceclor	Anti-infective	Eli Lilly and Co.	$ 640.00
9	Seldane	Antihistamine	Marion Merrell Dow Inc.	
10	Naprosyn	Antiarthritic/analgesic	Syntex Corp.	$ 609.80
11	Cipro	Anti-infective	Miles Inc.	
12	Capoten	Antihypertensive	Bristol-Myers Squibb Co.	$ 598.00
13	Xanax	Antianxiety medicine	The Upjohn Co.	$ 545.00
14	Epogen	Erythropoiesis enhancer	Amgen Inc.	$ 506.30
15	Premarin	Estrogen replacement therapy	Wyeth-Ayerst Labs	$ 505.00
16	Calan line	Antihypertensive/ antianginal	G.D. Searle & Co.	$ 452.00
17	**PEPCID**	Antiulcer agent	Merck & Co., Inc.	$ 440.00
18	Lopid	Cholesterol reducer	Warner-Lambert Co.	$ 427.00
19	Proventil	Bronchodilator	Schering-Plough Corp.	$ 426.00
20	Neupogen	Biological response modifier	Amgen Inc.	$ 422.20

Ginger's anti-ulcer properties pose a challenge to three of the twenty top-selling drugs in the U.S., Zantac, Tagamet and Pepcid. Sales for these drugs exceed $2.8 billion annually.[175]

rameters and (2) synergistic components.

To fully appreciate the decided advantage of ginger over H2-receptor antagonists, a look at how the two elements achieve their effect is necessary. The H2-receptor antagonist Tagamet is a convenient example because it is specifically compared with ginger in the research.

What ginger and Tagamet have in common is: (1) they reduce the total volume of gastric juices;[169-170,176] and (2) they possess ulcer-protective properties. By reducing total gastric volume, cimetidine and ginger clearly minimize the digestive tract's exposure to irritation. While cimetidine showed greater activity against "severe lesions," its impact on thc enzyme pepsin probably offsets this advantage.

An important difference between cimetidine and ginger arises in their respective effects on pepsin and pH. Pepsin is essential to split dietary protein into smaller molecules. For it to be active, however, the medium must be acidic. If gastric pH rises, or becomes less acidic, pepsin's activity decreases. In laboratory rats, cimetidine causes a 92 percent increase in pH to 4.2, while with ginger, the levels remain constant with controls at pH 2.3.[170]

Short and long term ramifications of an increased pH and less active pepsin, although seldom studied and as yet not verified, could potentially be quite significant. These include: compromised absorption of dietary protein, vitamin B_{12} and iron, and an increase in opportunistic infections of the digestive tract.[176]

"Whatever elements nature does not introduce in vegetables, the natural food of all animal life–directly of herbivorous, indirectly of carnivorous, are to be regarded with suspicion."

Oliver Wendell Holmes, 1861[177]

From Diarrhea to Constipation

ROOT NOTES

To call ginger "a digestive herb" is an understatement. In addition to enhancing digestion and protecting against ulcers and liver toxicity, ginger is found effective in treating both constipation and diarrhea.

From all parts of the world, virtually every ethnomedical text citing ginger lauds its benefits to digestion. A review of current scientific literature clearly shows substantiation for the thousands of years of empirical observation.

Ginger offers a diversity of digestive values which H2-receptor antagonists are simply incapable of providing. Included in this array of added benefits are enzyme-enhanced protein digestion,[67-69] digestive stimulation,[21,178-179] anti-diarrheal activity,[21] probiotic support,[180] liver protection[181] and anti-emetic[182-191] properties. Interestingly, known side effects of H2-receptor antagonists include diarrhea, nausea and hepatotoxicity,[192-193] problems which the consumption of ginger can actually address.

Ginger's enzyme action and digestive stimulation are direct synergists to its previously mentioned anti-ulcer effect. Even though ginger does not significantly affect pH or pepsin potency, it, like the H2-receptor antagonists, does reduce the gastric volume.

All who have experienced ginger as a digestive aid can attest that whatever digestive capacity is compromised by a reduction in gastric volume is well compensated for by other principal actions. These principal actions are undoubtedly those identified as the powerful protein-digesting enzyme and the digestive stimulant.

While enzymes promote protein digestion, stimulant actions increase bile secretion which will "facilitate absorption of fat and electrolytes." A side benefit of increased bile secretion will be relief of constipation and excretion of small gallstones.[21,178]

Another aspect of ginger which might have anti-ulcer synergy is its principal probiotic[70-72,180] and antitoxic actions. A new theory that is gaining recognition proposes that bacteria called Helicobacter pylori play a material role in the development of peptic ulcers.[116,194] Although there are no specific studies on ginger and this particular bacterial species, ginger has been shown to possess "sig-

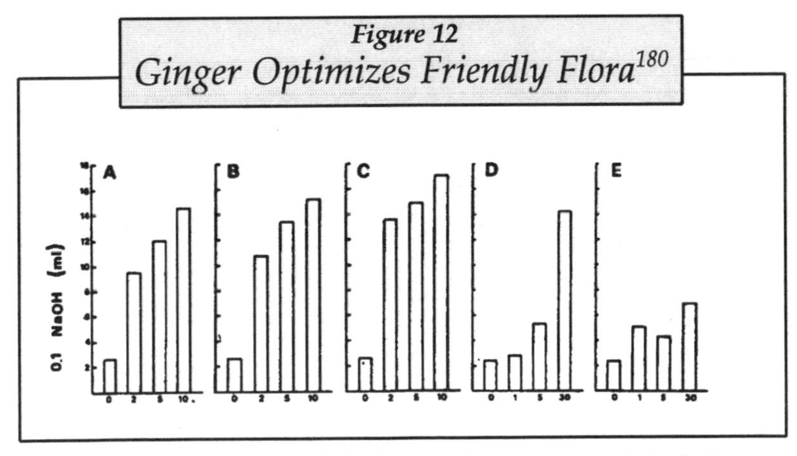

Figure 12
Ginger Optimizes Friendly Flora[180]

A= Pepper B=Cinnamon C=GINGER D=Garlic Powder E=Fresh Garlic Extract
When compared with all tested spices, ginger most encourages the growth of a "friendly" flora species, Lactobacillus plantarum. Remarkably, ginger is simultaneously antimicrobial against toxic bacteria like E. coli.

nificant activity" against a wide range of gram-negative and gram-positive bacteria. These include Escherichia coli, Proteus vulgaris, Salmonella typhimurium, Staphylococcus aureus and Streptococcus viridans.[180] Interestingly, while ginger is clearly inhibitory to these pathogenic species, it actually appears to stimulate the growth of potentially beneficial Lactobacillus species. Such is the wisdom of nature. *(See Figure 12.)*

How an Herbalist Spells Relief

☙ ROOT NOTES ❧

Nausea can range in severity from a simple symptom to a life-threatening complication of chemotherapy, surgery or pregnancy. Due to a remarkable series of chemical reactions, ginger is capable of alleviating this most unpleasant of physical experiences.

Of all ginger's effects, its antiemetic or antinausea property is probably the best known today. Thanks to the pioneer work of Daniel Mowrey published in the prestigious journal *Lancet*,[187] it is becoming increasingly common to see people taking ginger capsules on long car trips or boat rides. Although this work has met with recent controversy,[195-196] the body of research including both laboratory animal and human studies, strongly suggests that ginger is an effective aid to counter nausea and vomiting.

What Do Ocean Travel and Pregnancy Have in Common?

Whether nausea results from chemotherapy, ocean travel, pregnancy (see "Safety First" on page 50) or gynecological surgery, ginger is the treatment of choice.

It is reported that 90 percent of all patients receiving chemotherapy suffer from nausea and vomiting. At the University of Alabama in 1987 researchers reported "significant findings" concluding that patients who received additional ginger "reported less severity and duration of nausea."[183] The Alabama work was supported by a Japanese study in 1989 where researchers concluded that in laboratory animals ginger was "the first natural medicine to be reported to antagonize the profound emesis caused by a chemotherapeutic agent."[182]

When eighty naval cadets unaccustomed to sailing in heavy seas were studied to test the benefit of ginger, researchers concluded that without side effects "ginger root reduced the tendency to vomiting and cold sweating significantly better than placebo did."[186]

For the nausea of pregnancy ginger has offered many women relief from this most unpleasant of symptoms. Even the condition "hyperemesis gravidarum," a severe nausea which can complicate up to 50 percent of normal pregnancies, was eased by ginger. A double-blind randomized cross-over trial concluded that ginger scored "significantly greater" for relief of symptoms. When the women were asked their choices, 70.4 percent preferred ginger while only 29.6 percent had no preference or selected the placebo treatment.[191]

Lastly, ginger has been used successfully to treat the 30 percent incidence of serious nausea caused by major gynecological surgery. In sixty women who experienced this debilitating side effect, researchers found that there were "significantly fewer recorded incidences of nausea" with ginger than with the placebo and that ginger was comparable to the drug metoclopromide.[190,190a] An important note is that unlike ginger which has only positive benefits, metoclopromide has a long list of side effects including mental depression and tardive dyskenesia.[197]

The conflicting works of Wood and Stewart[195-196] to those of Mowrey and Grontved[187-188] suggest that the effectiveness of ginger in treating motion sickness might be dependent upon the specific type and duration of motion, length of prior consumption and freshness of product.

A Pause on Nausea

The anti-emetic property of ginger is a good example of how a plant's principal actions interplay to create an effect. Although nausea can result from many factors, the most common is if there is food in the stomach and rapid motion or stress is encountered. Obviously if food is in the stomach for a shorter period of time, there is less likelihood of nausea.◆

The two most obvious actions of ginger which might empty the stomach more quickly are its digestive enzyme and stimulant actions. Enzymes will catalyze the stomach's protein digestion while the stimulating volatile oils of ginger have been shown to enhance transport.[178]

Underlying these actions is another complex principal

◆ A recent study challenges the theory that ginger's anti-emetic effect is associated with enhanced gastric emptying.[196a]

action involving the balancing of a blood platelet-derived storage product called 5-HT (5-hydroxytryptamine) or serotonin. It has been reported that ginger modulates this amine,[154,179,182,198] explaining ginger's effectiveness in treating nausea as well as both constipation and diarrhea.

Interestingly, serotonin-balancing action has a broad range of added potential effects besides countering emesis including anti-inflammatory,[199] anti-ulcer,[200] anti-asthmatic,[201] normalizing blood pressure[202] and preventing potentially fatal cerebral vasospasms.[203-204] Not surprisingly, the first two effects of serotonin-balancing have already been demonstrated as benefits of ginger in the research.

Double Your Investment

ROOT NOTES

There is an old expression that you are what you eat. A more recent adaptation of this adage is you are what you absorb. Ginger holds a many thousand year reputation as being a "carrier" herb or an herb which enhances the absorption of other nutrients. This feature is pertinent or vital to people taking dietary supplements or who have weak digestive systems. Studies suggest that daily consumption of ginger might enhance nutrient absorption by as much as 200%.

Why has ginger been included in the majority of traditional remedies for thousands of years? The explanation given by traditional healers is that ginger acts as a "carrier" and improves the value of all other herbs in a formulation. Not surprisingly, modern research offers a justification for this empirical herbal observation.[8,205-206]

Attempting to understand the ancient Ayurvedic formulation technique which widely prescribed ginger and two other herbs, a group of Indian researchers studied one of these herbs and a constituent. The herb long pepper and its constituent piperine were examined for their effects on drug absorption. Long pepper and piperine improved absorption of two different drugs by 200 and 100 percent respectively.[8] Researchers concluded that a strong bioavailability justification was probable for the inclusion of long pepper, black pepper and ginger (referred to as "trikatu") in multiple formulations.

The researchers in the Indian study theorized a four-part mechanism for the effects of trikatu: "1) promoting absorption from the gastrointestinal tract, 2) protecting the drug from being metabolized/oxidized in the first passage through liver after being absorbed, 3) a combination of these two mechanisms, or 4) causing increased production of bile."

Considering that some of ginger's components appear to be in the blood for several days,[207] it is not farfetched to propose that ginger's bioavailability effect might be a sustained one. Since it is common knowledge that vitamins and minerals will have little value if they are not properly absorbed, a practical and more natural application of ginger's absorption-accelerating capabilities would be the inclusion of ginger in one's daily supplement program to enhance nutrient bioavailability.◆

"Ginger is generally combined with herbs going into the abdominal area, because it is a carrier. Ginger is an herb which accentuates so many herbs."

Dr. John Christopher[205]

◆ Interestingly, ginger is also recognized in the cosmetic industry as a transdermal drug accelerator.[206]

The Worms Crawl Out

ROOT NOTES

Although parasites are an unpleasant topic, it is unfortunately one which needs to be approached. Considering that 25 million Americans are potentially afflicted, a daily preventive and possible curative is definitely needed. Studies show that ginger is remarkably effective against some of the world's most dangerous parasites and, unlike virtually all antiparasitic medications, it is without negative side effects.

An important property of ginger which affects all systems, particularly the digestive, is its anthelmintic or antiparasitic effect.[39,73-81] The ramifications of this effect are more important than most people suspect. Jane Brody, a science writer for the *New York Times*, recently summarized the magnitude of this issue.[208]

> "Worms may be unthinkable in this cleanliness-obsessed society, yet an estimated 25 million Americans, many of them young children and many from middle class and affluent families, are often unknowing hosts to tiny intestinal worms."
>
> *Jane Brody*[208]

Brody's concern is echoed by other reputable sources which concur that "most available figures on the prevalence of parasitic infections in the U.S. are underestimates"[209] and that over one billion people in the world are "host to various types of worms."[210-211]

Clinical findings on ginger reveal that it possesses a

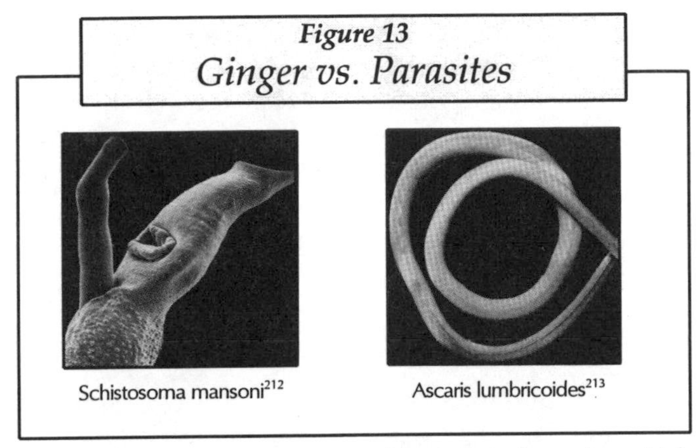

Schistosoma and Ascaris are two of the principal parasites which collectively infect billions of people worldwide. Promising research indicates that ginger can inhibit or kill these dangerous parasites.

Reprinted with permission from "Medical Parasitology" by E.K. Markell, M. Voge, D.T. John, W.B. Saunders Co., Philadelphia, 1986.

---

broad range of anthelmintic effects including activity against some of the world's most prevalent and dangerous parasites. *(See Figure 13.)* This strong activity has been demonstrated with nematodes or roundworms including Anisakis, Ascaris and Filaria and trematodes or flatworms in the Schistosoma genus. Although most of this work is performed using in vitro tests, the results are promising and deserve further study.

Ginger's anthelmintic effect is probably a consequence of a combination of principal actions including those which involve potent enzymes and pungent stimulants. A brief summary of the work follows.

- Anisakis, which is principally acquired through the consumption of sushi or raw fish, is an important parasitic infection in Japan which is increasing "markedly" in the U.S.[73] Although the exact number of cases is unclear, no effective drug treatment exists to eliminate the worms which typically become embedded in the stomach or bowel wall. Extracts of ginger and two of its constituents caused more than 90 percent of the larvae to lose spontaneous movement within four hours and to be destroyed completely within sixteen hours. Interestingly, pyrantel pamoate, an antinematodal drug, had no lethal effect even at a relatively high concentration. Not surprisingly, ginger is traditionally eaten with sushi in Japan.

- Ascaris lumbricoides which is lethal to approximately 20,000 people annually and affects an estimated one billion people worldwide, was effectively inhibited by ginger extract.[211,214]
- Filariae, which affect at least 80 million people worldwide,[215] were effectively reduced in dogs by an extract of ginger by approximately 98 percent without any reported toxic effects.[75]
- Schistosoma, which is becoming increasingly prevalent in the U.S.,[216] is considered the second major parasitic disease in the world.[217] This infection is particularly insidious in that the parasite is capable of ingesting as many as 330,000 red blood cells per hour in a laboratory mouse.[218] Ginger "completely abolished" the infectivity[39] in its early phases and in young children ginger extract was found to significantly reduce the egg count in the urine indicating a systemic action.[79]

The Common Cold Meets Its Match

☙ ROOT NOTES ❧

The common cold has undoubtedly been a disagreeable aspect of the human experience since the beginning of recorded history. From the earliest written records to the conclusions of nearly 25,000 early 20th century physicians, ginger has been recognized as an herb of choice for lessening the severity of a cold.

The Danish researcher Srivastava, whose pioneering work established ginger as a powerful therapeutic tool for arthritis treatment, observed a "side effect" of ginger consumption that has been confirmed throughout the most ancient traditions of medicine.

While Srivastava's patients reported a reduction in pain from arthritis, they also observed that they contracted fewer or less severe colds or infections.[89] The same observations have been made from the historic works of Ayurveda to the writings of the U.S. eclectic physicians of the early 20th century, Felter and Lloyd.

As with many of ginger's observed effects, a blend of principal actions is probably responsible for its cold-fighting properties. These include its eicosanoid balance, cytoprotection, and probiotic principal actions. Undoubtedly, its antitoxic principal action, with distinct antibacterial, antiviral,[219] antifungal[220-222] and antihistaminic observed effects, is also at play.[223]

Getting at the Roots of Cancer

☙ ROOT NOTES ❧

It is widely believed that environmental exposure to toxins is responsible for as many as 80% of all cancers.[223a] When tested against two accepted standards for toxicity, ginger significantly reduced their life-threatening potential.

We are exposed to an endless variety of toxins in our air, water and food. The degree to which we are able to adapt to and detoxify these agents will to a major extent determine our quality of life and longevity. Benzo(a)pyrene and pyrolysis products (burnt byproducts) of the amino acid tryptophan, commonly referred to as Trp-P, are considered laboratory standards for creating toxicity. Trp-P is generally regarded to have a higher mutagenic or cancer-causing potential than benzo(a)pyrene.[224]

Ginger and a number of its constituents "showed remarkable effects"[228] and were antimutagenic to both benzo(a)pyrene and (Trp-P).[◆9,224-229]

There are only a few references in the scientific literature investigating ginger's anticancer effects but the results warrant further research.[□231-233] In vitro tests suggest

◆ Another testament to ginger's protective values is that animals dosed with ginger as close as five minutes prior to irradiation experienced a significantly increased survival rate.[230]

□ Recent research suggesting that the prostaglandin-inhibiting properties of aspirin "block" a colon tumor's growth factors, opens another field for the potential anticancer benefits of ginger.[233a]

ginger is cytotoxic to tumor cells and extract of ginger will extend the lifespan of laboratory animals induced with Dalton's lymphoma ascites and Ehrlich ascites tumors by 11 percent.[231] To achieve its effect, it appears that ginger functions from the most fundamental levels of the immune system by inducing neutrophils which, according to a recent report, can explain why ginger might "stimulate host resistance against various diseases."[234]

The True Meaning of Synergy

Interestingly, some of ginger's most active elements included in the broad class of gingerols and shogaols are potentially mutagenic.[225,229] It is only when other constituents like zingerone are reintroduced into the system that the mutagenicity is suppressed or actually reversed.

This research on mutagenicity is justification for being wary of isolating active plant compounds. Considering that a minimum of 25 percent of all modern drugs are plant derived and that these compounds are achieved through isolation, this point is an important one.

Within the matrix of ginger's minimum 300 compounds, one can only ponder the significance of one constituent to the whole effect. Further, the cliché of trying to manipulate or fool nature is an image that probably has particular significance when attempting to isolate and deliver an herb's so-called active agent.

All Systems Go

☙ ROOT NOTES ❧

It is a somewhat foreign concept in the era of modern medicine's "magic bullets" to imagine that a single food or herb could benefit every part of the body. However, just as sleep leaves the entire body refreshed, ginger is capable of invigorating and balancing a wide range of body systems. Ginger's life-supporting effects are noted from the circulatory and respiratory systems to the reproductive organs.

A term that is now being widely used in alternative medicine, particularly to describe the action of certain herbs, is "adaptogenic." An herb's adaptogenic action is believed responsible for increasing "non-specific" resistance of an organism to adverse influences. Although this principal action is somewhat nebulous, it does help explain numerous observed effects of herbs such as their balancing of system parameters like blood pressure and cholesterol.

Under the umbrella of ginger's adaptogenic principal action is its ability to normalize blood sugar[72] and cholesterol,[235-237] while stimulating or toning the circulatory,[238-241] respiratory,[155,238,242] and reproductive[243-246] systems.

In laboratory animals, ginger or its constituents reduced artificially elevated glucose levels by 51 percent, significantly lowered chemically induced hypercholesteremia, positively affected heart muscle action and exhibited "an intense antitussive effect in comparison with dihydrocodeine phosphate."[155]

Although there are no studies to confirm the historical observation that ginger might possess aphrodisiac properties, Joshua Backon, a researcher who has published a number of articles on ginger, suggests that ginger holds potential as a tool against impotence due to its ability to inhibit thromboxane synthetase.[243] Dr. Backon also proposes the same mechanism might be behind ginger's ability to relieve menstrual cramping and discomfort.[244]

On a side note, ginger is used externally by traditional Oriental practitioners to affect a number of body systems. Most thought provoking of this research is a recent Chinese report on breech births. The study indicated that simply applying a ginger paste to a specific "acupressure" point in these pregnant women[246] allowed a 77.4 percent correction rate as opposed to the control group which had only a 51.6 percent correction rate.[81] Whatever the underlying reason for the correction of breech position "effect," it is clear that applying a ginger-based transdermal cream or paste to acupressure points may have added benefits.

5

Give Me My Ginger

Safety First

"During the 2.5 year period of ginger consumption, no side effects were reported."

K.C. Srivastava[89]

The multi-milennia safety record of ginger is one of its most valuable testimonials. The historical literature contains virtually no mention of adverse effects and the body of modern scientific literature reports a unanimous "no side effect."[32,89-90,170,185-186,191] As appealing as it might be to say that there is no limit to daily ginger dosage, especially in light of the 50 gram dosages consumed in some studies with no side effects and its historically liberal consumption even as a vegetable, common sense dictates that upper limits must exist.

In attempting to define an upper or safety limit for ginger, there are two areas which at least justify mention and possible prudence. Keep in mind that what is mentioned below is theoretical and there are no specific studies to support these concerns.

Since ginger is a modulator of eicosanoids and can specifically inhibit thromboxane synthetase, Joshua Backon alerts regular consumers that blood-clotting times after surgery might be affected. Backon specifically raises this concern before "wholeheartedly" endorsing ginger supplementation for nausea after gynecological surgery.

The other related reservation regarding ginger is consumption during pregnancy, specifically in the first trimester. Ginger has historically been used as an emmenagogue and in large doses as an abortifacient, although in the latter case the dosage is not clearly defined. If one balances this historical application with research findings that ginger is statistically effective and safe for the nausea of pregnancy,[191] my conclusion is that moderation should be exercised.

As a conservative safety guideline during the first trimester and before parturition, it is advised that dosages used in the Fischer-Rasmussen study (1000 mg. powdered root or 2 teaspoons of ginger syrup per day) should not be exceeded.

Regarding lactation, one source reports that it is well known in Jamaica that ginger can reduce a lactating mother's milk flow.[247] This can be either a benefit or a detriment depending on the desire of the mother.

"Some of the patients with arthritic disorders who mistakenly took 3-4 times, or even more, the dose (0.5-1.0 gram powdered ginger/day) suggested by us, reported quicker and better [arthritis] relief than those on the recommended dose."

K.C. Srivastava[89]

Is More Better?

Taking into consideration the body of ginger research, a broad and safe guideline for the general population to gain the preventive benefits of ginger is a daily recommended intake of a minimum of 1200 mg. of the root powder (capsules), 90 drops of extract or two teaspoons of the syrup. There is obviously great flexibility in the safety ranges for incorporating more liberal amounts of ginger into the diet.

I have heard from some people who have taken doses of ginger larger than that recommended above that ginger can actually upset the stomach. To avoid this, an important common sense suggestion, regardless of the dosage, is to increase dietary intake of ginger gradually. This is especially important for people with sensitive stomachs or ulcerative conditions.

Using therapeutic or larger doses of ginger as part of a disease treatment program is a process which would best be guided by the patient's holistic health practitioner. This is noted because in large doses ginger might affect the bioavailability of other therapeutic aids and either intensify or negate aspects of the prescribed medication's effectiveness.

When working on a therapeutic program with your practitioner, consider the daily dosage and observation of benefits mentioned in the Srivastava studies. The dosage which delivered the antiarthritic benefits without side effects was approximately 3 to 7 grams and some of the most dramatic results were noted when

Figure 14
What You Don't Want with Your Ginger

Commercial Functions	**Chemical Compound**
Insecticides	Navan
Mercury Compounds	Ceresan
Chlorinated Hydrocarbons	Demosan, Diflotan, DDT
Fungicides	Bavistin, Dithane m-45, Kitazin
Fumigants	Ethylene oxide

The above compounds are a sampling of chemicals to which commercial ginger can be exposed. To avoid these potentially toxic chemicals, it is highly recommended that one request organic certification before purchasing a ginger supplement.

doses were significantly higher, reaching upwards of 50 grams daily.◆

If ginger is used as an analgesic, consider that benefits range from immediate to as long as 1-3 months for more chronic conditions. If it does take longer to observe the benefits of ginger, it is reassuring to know that, while one system is being healed, others are likewise being balanced. No modern drug can make this claim so confidently or safely.

◆ Regarding an accurate determination of therapeutic dosages, I appeal to the medical profession to help set these standards by embracing the potential of ginger through research and application.

Quality Is Everything

The first concern for those who supplement their diet with ginger should be the quality of the original root. Ginger can be valuable in many forms: fresh, as a dried powder, syrup, extract or in capsules. However, if the original material is old, shriveled, moldy or chemically treated, it will obviously not yield the same values as a product created from fresh organically grown roots.

Beginning with fresh root as opposed to dry powder is an important advantage for a quality product because root quality can be evaluated. Starting with even a fresh plant though has its limitations. The most obvious one is that commercial roots are often barraged with chemicals, including mercury compounds, chlorinated hydrocarbons, fungicides and fumigants, during processing and storage.[248-252] *(See Figure 14.)*

To Each Her Own

Fresh or Dry?

The question of which finished form of ginger is best, fresh, dry, syrup, capsule or extract, cannot be easily answered. It is fair to say that each form has distinct advantages and that a combination of products is probably best. The modulation of two principal ginger constituent groups, the gingerols and shogaols, is an example supporting this claim. It is widely accepted that gingerols convert to shogaols upon drying.

Gingerols and shogaols each have their own advantages. For example, gingerols are more potent as antihepatotoxics[181] and anthelmintics,[39] while shogaols appear to be more effective as antipyretics and analgesics.[155,155a]

Another noteworthy point to cloud the issue is the clinical finding that roasted ginger, commonly used in the Orient for digestive problems, may have distinct advantages over dried ginger in preventing ulcers.[167]

One Chinese study suggests, however, that all the forms have more in common than one would suspect. Of 25 studied elements, there was only a maximum variation of three novel or missing elements.[253]

Get Fresh!

Whatever the final form, it is easy to argue that there is an intangible advantage to the fresh root. The flavor of fresh ginger is itself a study in culinary art.◆ This is underlined by a recent fragrance test which noted that fresh ginger can be recognized for its scent at a dilution as low as 1 part in 35,000, while powdered ginger is only 1 part in 1500-2000.[254]

The fresh form can be used in many applications including compresses, as a tea and in cooking. Grate fresh rhizome (root) and use as desired.

A small amount of fresh ginger juice also accentuates the powerful health values of carrot juice. Add the juice gradually to your routine as it is quite potent.

◆ Figure 15 demonstrates the extent of worldwide interest in the flavor of ginger.

Certainly the Sweetest

A honey-based syrup has traditionally been used to deliver the benefits of herbs. The properties of honey offer excellent synergistic values to ginger, especially when the dry and fresh constituents of ginger are low-heat-infused into the honey. Besides enhancing flavor, preservation, and the variety of applications for a ginger prod-

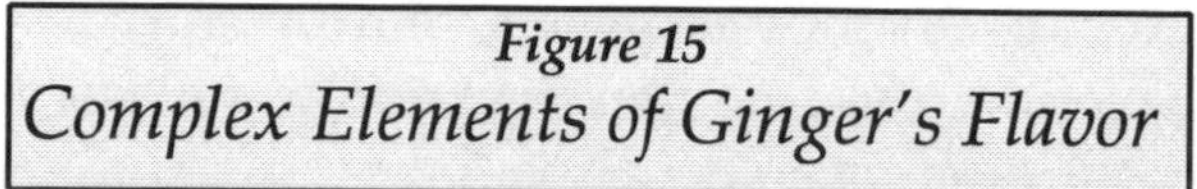

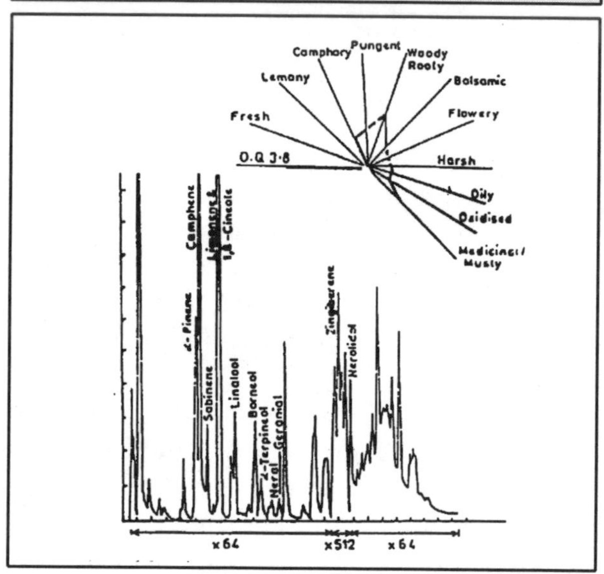

The flavor of ginger has been extensively studied throughout the world. The two images above, presented in "CRC Critical Reviews," each delineate particular aspects of what gives ginger its distinctive flavor. The top image is a subjective taste rating score associated with the lower gas chromatogram. When the two are combined a signature profile can be given to a ginger sample.[255]

uct, honey possesses its own range of antibacterial,[256-258] anticancer,[259] antifungal,[260-261] wound healing,[262-268] and antiulcer[269-271] properties. A book similar to this one could easily be written on honey itself, but a few points deserve mention here in conjunction with ginger.

While honey broadens ginger's antibacterial and antifungal benefits, honey combined with ginger presents an even more effective peptic ulcer formulation. Honey is protective to the gastric mucosa[270] and shows significant activity against Helicobacter pylori,[269] the species associated with peptic ulcers. For people with blood-sugar problems, evidence suggests that honey is significantly better tolerated than commonly used simple sugars like sucrose.[272-275] A factor in honey is also found active against candida albicans.[276]

In addition to using ginger and honey as a health syrup, this combination can be used as a hot beverage or tea sweetener, cooking seasoning or table sauce, dessert topping or mixed with carbonated water to create a delicious homemade ginger ale.

One to three teaspoons daily is a general dosage guideline.

"Sweet route to heading off colon cancer"

"In recent years, a host of studies have identified a broad spectrum of medical attributes in honey–including antifungal, antibacterial, anti-inflammatory, antiproliferative, and cancer-drug-potentiating properties. Now, researchers at the American Health Foundation in Valhalla, N.Y., have uncovered another. In the September 15 *Cancer Research*, Bandaru S. Reddy and his co-workers describe the ability of honey-derived caffeic esters to inhibit the development of precancerous changes in the colon of rats given a known carcinogen. These esters come from the propolis–the brown, resinous, tree-derived material that honeybees use to cement together their hives. Reddy's group considers three derivatives of the caffeic esters promising enough to use in the longer-term animal studies of colon cancer."

Science News 1993 [277]

From Tablespoon to Tub

After the quality source has been verified, powdered ginger can be effectively used in a variety of ways. For its rubefacient, stimulating, transdermal and aromatherapeutic effects, ginger powder is excellent as a moistened chest compress *(see Figure 16)* or added by the tablespoon to a hot bath for relief of cold symptoms.

Powdered ginger can also be formed into a paste with water or herbal tea for external applications in treating sprains or headaches.

Ginger capsules allow dried powdered ginger to be conveniently and healthfully added to the diet as part of a supplement or treatment regime.

Figure 16

Dr. Koji Yamoda's Ginger Compress

While bringing a gallon of distilled or spring water to boil in a large, lidded enamel pot, wash 1-1/2 fresh, unpeeled ginger root and grate by hand using a rotating, clockwise motion. This keeps tough fibers from building up on the grater.

Place the grated ginger in a clean muslin cloth, slightly moistened, and tie at top to form a bag, leaving room inside for air and water to circulate.

Before dropping this bag into the pot, gently squeeze the juice from the bag into the water which should no longer be boiling.

Cover pot and simmer for 7 minutes.

The resulting liquid should have a golden hue and a distinctive ginger aroma.

When ready, remove pot from stove and set aside.

When the liquid is still hot but not scalding, dip a terry cloth hand towel and apply directly to site of pain.

The compress should be kept fairly warm for 15 to 20 minutes and repeat again 4 to 6 hours later.

This remedy of Dr. Yamoda is said to relieve a wide variety of external and internal pains including neuralgia, stiffness, swollen glands and toothache. A ginger compress is reported to be effective for patients suffering from asthma and bronchitis. Consult with your holistic physician when treating serious disorders.[278]

Alcohol's Bright Side

Alcohol is recognized traditionally and in modern research as the best extraction agent for the properties of most herbs. A double-macerated or highly concentrated alcohol extract of dried ginger can also serve as a natural preservative-base for the freshly extracted juice of organic ginger. The addition of juice provides a dual purpose; it adds the full enzyme value of fresh ginger while lowering the final alcohol concentration to a level that most people should well tolerate.

> "Alcohol and acetone have been generally used for extraction of the [ginger] oleoresin. Both solvents give satisfactory oleoresins although the yield with alcohol is reported to be higher, in some cases as much as three times."
>
> *V.S. Govindarajan* [279]

The principal benefits of the extracted form are concentration and convenience. Easily portable, 30 to 90 drops taken throughout the day can deliver the most active and concentrated benefits of ginger.*

* As an interesting side note, it is a traditional practice in the Middle East and particularly Saudi Arabia to add ginger to coffee. I have heard from coffee drinkers here in the U.S. that by doing this they require less coffee to deliver its stimulating properties. Considering ginger's principal stimulant and bioavailability actions, these observed effects are not surprising.

To mix ginger with coffee, one can simply add powdered or fresh grated ginger into the preperked coffee grounds. An alternative would be to add the alcohol extract described above to the already brewed coffee. I offer this simply as a point of information and not as an endorsement of coffee drinking.

Figure 17
Heinerman on Ginger

ABDOMINAL CRAMPS	Equal parts of Ginger and Hop tea
BLOOD CIRCULATION	Warm tea
BLOOD CLOT	Powdered Ginger (capsules) or Ginger tea
CAPSICUM SUBSTITUTE	Action similar to Cayenne pepper
CHEST (heart pains)	Tea.
CHICKENPOX	Warm Ginger tea
COLITIS	Ginger tea, capsules, or warm Ginger enema
DIARRHEA	As a tea
HEADACHE	1 cup cool tea
HYPOGLYCEMIA	Generally 3-5 capsules a day without Licorice; 2 per day with Licorice
INDIGESTION	Capsules or tea
INFECTION	Capsules, tea or enema
LARYNGITIS	Hot Ginger tea with honey and lemon juice
LUNG CONGESTION (asthma; bronchitis; common cold; cough; hoarseness; influenza)	Warm tea
LYMPH GLAND CLEANSER	As a tea
MEASLES	Tea, capsules or enema
MENSTRUATION (to promote)	Warm tea
MILD PARALYSIS (shock)	Chew a little of the grated root for mouth and tongue paralysis
MUMPS	See measles
PERSPIRATION (to promote)	Warm tea
SALIVA	Stimulates the flow of it; good for digestive disorders
SCIATICA	Warm tea. Rubdown with Ginger oil. Warm Ginger packs on site of pain and stiffness
STREP THROAT (sore throat; tonsillitis)	Chew the rootstock
URINATION (to promote)	Tea
WEAKNESS	Warm tea or capsules
WOUNDS	Wash with Ginger tea. Take capsules internally.

The applications of ginger are virtually endless. John Heinerman is a noted researcher who has written numerous articles and texts on herbs. Heinerman's suggested uses for ginger are included here to exemplify a few of these applications.[280]

6

Freedom & Health at the Crossroads

"The Task Force (FDA) considered many issues in its deliberations including to insure that the existence of dietary supplements (vitamins, minerals, amino acids, herbs and other) on the market does not act as a disincentive for drug development."

FDA Task Force Report released June 15, 1993[281]

"We don't know what we're doing in medicine....Perhaps one quarter to one-third of medical services may be of little or no benefit to patients."

Dr. David Eddy, Director, Duke U. Health Policy Research[282]

"If you're feeling well, just stay away from the doctor."

Eugene Robbins, M.D., Professor Emeritus, Stanford University[283]

"The health-care system is in crisis, if not chaos. If you really want to beat the system, don't use it."

C. Everett Koop, M.D., Former U.S. Surgeon General[284]

Death by Prescription

More than 50 percent of the average American diet consists of processed foods, containing some 3,000 different food additives. The typical American ingests 15 pounds of these food additives each year.[285] Every hour 660,000 animals are killed for meat in the United States,[286] and every three days the average American consumes a pound of white sugar. In 1982, the National Research Council determined that diet was "probably the greatest single factor in the epidemic of cancer particularly for cancers of the breast, colon and prostate."[287]

The current prevailing health-care system is unfortunately incapable of changing this direction. Instead of remedying the underlying reasons why so many of us are sick, the system is structured to simply bandage the problem or manage disease.

Studies show that we don't need more doctors or more physicals. The Kaiser Permanente Health Group in California reported no significant difference in death rates for people who did or did not receive physicals.[288]

We certainly don't need more surgery. More harm than good has been demonstrated by many commonly performed procedures. For example, men who receive radical prostate surgery experience incontinence and impotence rates from the surgery itself of 30 and 90 percent respectively, while men who avoid this surgical procedure are found to benefit more from "watchful waiting." The researcher Dr. John Wasson concluded in the study published in the *Journal of the American Medical Association* (JAMA) that, "We have, in essence, an epidemic of treatment and no scientific proof that it's valid...The take-home message is that we don't know what we're doing, but we're doing a lot of it."[289]

Lastly, no one really believes we need more prescription drugs. By the time we Americans are age 50, one out of three of us will be on eight or more prescription drugs[290] and according to recent figures cited in JAMA, between 60,000 to 140,000 of us will die each year from adverse reactions to these drugs.[291]

> "51.5 percent of drugs approved by FDA have serious post approval risks including heart failure, birth defects, kidney failure, blindness and convulsions."
>
> *1990 GAO Report*[292]

The Money Pit

To add irony to this macabre health scenario, our current "disease care" system is killing us financially.

Our total "health-care" bill is a staggering $3 billion daily, the highest of all industrialized nations. Included in this bill is an excessive 800 percent markup for the pharmaceutical industry's adverse-effect-riddled drugs.

The consequences of maintaining this system are already devastating to business and middle-class America. Health-care costs are the leading reason for bankruptcy and one million Americans earning $25,000-50,000 annually lost their health insurance last year alone due to inflated premium costs.[293]

Recognizing the peril of this crisis at a recent conference on health care, President Clinton banged a table with his fist and told the 300 participants that the cost of health care "...is a joke. It is going to bankrupt this country."[294]

Considering the tragic fact that among industrialized nations we place close to the lowest in life expectancy (15th) and highest in all cancer and heart disease rates, it is painfully obvious that our national health "system" is terribly ill, not to mention a very bad investment.

Milligrams of Hope

While we are getting poorer and probably sicker as a nation, there are flickers of hope. New doors are beginning to open in the renowned edifices of the U.S. healthcare establishment.

The most respected U.S. medical journals are now acknowledging that simple changes in diet and the mere addition of literally milligrams of dietary supplements can drastically improve the nation's health. Recently published studies proclaim that we can conceivably disarm two of our greatest killers, heart disease and cancer, by simply adding daily natural supplements of food constituents like antioxidants beta carotene and vitamin E to the diet.

Researchers are going so far as to declare that Americans supplementing their diets can "lower their risk of heart disease, independent of other risk factors for heart disease by as much as 40 to 50 percent."[292,295-296] Noting that heart attacks alone kill 600,000 Americans annually, this safe and easy type of prescription could potentially save hundreds of thousands of lives not to mention billions of dollars each year.

Considering that vitamins and other more powerful antioxidants naturally occur in certain herbs,[103-105,297-299] the profound untapped potential of dietary herbal supplements may soon be realized. Research around the world on readily available and inexpensive botanicals like ginger is mounting and even proving therapeutic potentials transcending those of our most powerful drugs.[300-304]

Lastly, the recent opening of the Office of Alternative Medicine (OAM) at the National Institutes of Health (NIH) rates perhaps as the most positive development. It is hard to believe that the NIH, a bastion of conservative allopathic medicine, has actually opened an office to examine the efficacy of alternative forms of health care like herbal medicine and acupuncture. Although the budget for this office is only one-five-thousandth of that of NIH as a whole, it is a promising sign of events to come.

The Roadblocks

Alternative health-care practitioners, herbs like ginger and other dietary supplements will never be fully appreciated or allowed to fulfill their mission unless major problems are identified and eradicated in our current health-care system. Needless to say, whole books are written trying to diagnose and answer these problems. Since the focus of this book is on ginger and not the intricacies of our current health-care establishment, this discussion will be very brief. Acknowledging the risk of being oversimplistic, there will hopefully be some value in the short solutions which are posed.

I would not be so foolish or unrealistic as to suggest eliminating the doctors or the drugs or the governmental establishment that has evolved to support them. Rather I would like to propound just a few aspects of these modern icons which I label as the roadblocks and propose the simplest of solutions.

The FDA

"The American public does not have the knowledge to make wise health-care decisions....Trust us. We will tell you what's good for you..."

David Kessler, FDA Commissioner on "Larry King Live," 1992[305]

The Problem

The agency given the authority to dictate what information is disseminated to the public on food, drugs and general health claims–the U.S. Food and Drug Administration (FDA)–has held a long bias against preventive health and the natural foods and dietary supplement industry.

The agency continues to further the notion that herbs and other dietary supplements are inherently dangerous. It refers to safe and soothing teas made with herbs like chamomile as "unknown brews" with dangers lurking within. *The FDA Consumer*, the agency journal, absurdly depicts herbal teas with a skull and crossbones.[306]

Considering that "three of the top four causes of lethal poisonings in the U.S. are FDA-approved drugs"[307] and that a toxicity category is virtually nonexistent for herbal dietary supplements, the "skull and crossbones" symbol is clearly misplaced.

To make matters worse, the agency has for the past 20 years continuously attempted through wily, circuitous and one-dimensional arguments to regulate virtually all traditional medicinal or tonic herbs out of the U.S. marketplace, threatening both national health and medical freedom of choice.

"Some so-called dietary supplement products that have no recognized nutritional role are sold for therapeutic uses. It is a simple fact that these products (herbs) are legally drugs and properly regulated as such."

Michael R. Taylor, FDA Deputy Commissioner of Policy[308]

☼The Solution☼

The government agency should appoint a panel of experts who are open-minded and aware of alternative health-care modalities. Fair and clear guidelines should be given, actually encouraging the use of safe and inexpensive dietary supplements and traditional medicines. Also, the structure of the process which results in drug companies spending up to $359 million for drug approval and marketing should be reevaluated.

The Pharmaceutical Industry

"In 1990 the top ten pharmaceutical houses had profit margins 3X that of the average Fortune 500 company...Over the past decade drug prices have risen almost triple the rate of inflation."

1990 GAO (General Accounting Office) report[309]

💣The Problem💣

The pharmaceutical industry is arguably the most serious obstacle to progress in our health-care system. Being the most greedy and profit-oriented segment, it will therefore be the hardest to change.

As difficult as it is to defend this industry, part of its problem lies in the regulatory structure for drug approval and the bloated $359 million it costs to develop and market drugs. These enormous expenses drive prices into the stratosphere and foster greed.

The most frightening aspect of the pharmaceutical industry however is its relationship with the nation's health-care providers, our medical doctors and its regulatory agency, the FDA.

In the millions of dollars behind each drug lies regulatory jobs at the FDA and a $5000 promotional allowance for the nation's 479,000 doctors.[282] In an exposé published in *Time* magazine some of these benefits to physicians were detailed such as Wyeth Ayerst's offering to doctors of 1000 points towards American Airlines travel for each patient put on the hypertension drug Inderal, and Ciba-Geigy's free Caribbean vacation for doctors sitting in on lectures on Estraderm.[310]

✡The Solution✡

The only way change will occur in this industry is through consumer awareness and diligence on the part of medical ethicists. Government should offer incentives for drug companies to develop less expensive, safer and more natural medications.

The Food Industry

"Among life's great dichotomies: Kids like junk food, but their parents want them to eat right. The folks behind the food are betting the kids win out...Companies are appealing to a fertile audience: Children ages 6 to 14 spend $7.3 billion a year and influence family buying of more than $120 billion a year."[311]

Selina Guber, President, Children's Market Research Inc.,

The Problem

How will we ever be healthy if our food is laden with chemicals and depleted of its life-giving values?

The problem with the food industry is epitomized in the above statement by Selina Guber.

The Solution

The food industry is driven by market forces. Increased pressure by consumer groups should continue to force product development of healthier food choices.

The Medical Establishment

"We've developed a medical system of specialists, who do ordinary things at very special prices."

C. Everett Koop, M.D., Former U.S. Surgeon General[311a]

The Problem

Perhaps the most serious problem with the medical profession is highlighted in the following combination of facts.[312]

1) Six of the ten leading causes of death among Americans are diet related including heart disease, cancer, stroke, diabetes mellitus, chronic liver disease and atherosclerosis.

2) Data from the Association of the American

Medical Colleges concludes that "In 1992, only one-fourth of the 127 medical schools in the United States taught nutrition as a required course." The number of medical schools with a required course in nutrition has actually decreased in recent years.

☼The Solution☼

A drastic and immediate change should be called for in the structure of medical education in the United States. How can our health-care providers truly help us if they can never really understand the problem?

The Insurance Industry

The insurance industry has driven the nation "to the brink of bankruptcy...It is time for all Americans to stand up and say to the insurance industry 'Enough is enough. We want our health care system back.' "

Hillary Rodham Clinton[313]

The Problem

Premiums for health insurance are like a spider's web directly tied into the escalating costs of medical technology. Not only can fewer and fewer Americans afford health insurance but even those with insurance find that when it is finally needed for a catastrophic illness, their coverage has been dropped through a loophole or technicality. Instead of dealing with the roots of why so many of us are sick, a large segment of the insurance industry has chosen to simply adapt by raising premiums and dropping coverage. Sadly, the industry actually denies reimbursement for lower-cost alternative health care treatments that are defined as "experimental."

☼The Solution☼

Insurance companies started on the right track when they reduced premiums for non-smokers. What about people who eat a whole food diet, exercise, practice stress reduction or take dietary supplements? Also, why should a drug treatment for ulcers be reimbursed at $100 while a $10 alternative ginger treatment be disallowed? The insurance companies could at least offer the choice.

Ginger Accepts the Challenge

One of the principal reasons I have chosen to write about ginger, besides my personal attraction to the herb, is its potential as a catalyst for positive change.

Ginger by its very existence can safely, inexpensively and successfully challenge the foundations of some of the giants of the pharmaceutical industry and many of their flagship products totaling literally billions of dollars in annual sales.

Ginger can also represent to the consumer a daily health and disease-preventive tonic with the added "side effect" of being a superior potential treatment for ulcers and inflammatory conditions.

And lastly because ginger rests virtually unrecognized in everyone's spice cabinet, it holds the promise of awakening consumer awareness to the vast potential herbs possess, a potential that can quite literally save our lives.

7

The Essence of Ginger

27 Main Points

Beyond Sisyphus

1. Ginger offers a variety of therapeutic effects which no modern drug can rival. Unfortunately, due to a monopolistic health-care system and an historically biased regulatory environment, full awareness of ginger's value has been limited *(pg. 1)*.

The Roots of Ginger

2. Ginger is the most popular of hundreds of members of the Zingiberaceae family. It requires tropical conditions and fertile soil for optimal growth *(pg. 4)*.

3. Over a period of 5,000 years, ginger traveled from Southeast Asia to the New World. Its trade helped shape the fate of many nations. In ancient cultures like India, ginger was revered as *vishwabhesaj* or "the universal medicine" *(pg. 5)*.

4. More than 25,000 physicians in the early part of the 20th century in the U.S., called the "eclectics," lauded the healing values of ginger *(pg. 6)*.

5. Ginger was used historically in different regions of the world for the same basic therapeutic values. These include: analgesic, antiarthritic, wound healing, anthelmintic, antiulcer, stimulant and aphrodisiac properties and for the treatment of a variety of respiratory, reproductive and digestive complaints. *(pg. 8)*.

Eicosanoids & Other Light Subjects

6. The "observed effects" of ginger are the result of the interactions of more than 300 constituents. The most well known of these are a group of compounds called gingerols and shogaols *(pg. 11)*.

7. When a combination of ginger's individual constituents interact in a therapeutically defined fashion, the combined activity is referred to as a "principal action" *(pg. 12)*.

8. A principal action can have many observed effects. Observed effects like anti-inflammatory, antiparasitic, antimicrobial and digestive can all result from ginger's principal enzyme action *(pg. 12)*.

9. An observed effect or benefit can also have a variety of principal actions at its roots. Various principal actions including enzyme, eicosanoid balance and antioxidant all can participate in ginger's anti-inflammatory effect *(pg. 13)*.

10. The key to understanding ginger is to appreciate the actions of substances called eicosanoids. Eicosanoids are physiologically active compounds which the body synthesizes from essential fatty acids. When

these elements become imbalanced, an amazing variety of disease conditions can evolve *(pg. 16)*.

11. The pharmaceutical industry has attempted to modulate eicosanoids to treat a host of disease conditions but has essentially failed because of serious side effects *(pg. 19)*.

12. Ginger naturally helps balance the vitally important eicosanoids without side effects *(pg. 20)*.

Ginger: The Healer

13. Intriguing studies by Danish rescarcher Srivastava and others illustrate ginger's therapeutic potential against arthritis. Ginger as a treatment modality offers many advantages over currently popular nonsteroidal anti-inflammatory drugs. Over a period of three to six months, clinical trials suggest that ginger is more effective than these commonly prescribed drugs and without serious side effects *(pg. 24)*.

14. Ginger has a critical application in the treatment of cardiovascular disorders. Like aspirin it can prevent thousands of deaths from heart attacks and strokes as well as colon cancer but unlike aspirin it will have no side effects *(pg. 26)*.

15. Ginger is a potent antiulcer treatment rivaling three of the nation's most popular drugs which account for $2.8 billion in sales annually *(pg. 31)*.

16. The antiulcer effect of ginger is complemented with a host of other important digestive values which include relief of both diarrhea and constipation, liver protection and probiotic support *(pg. 34)*.

17. The antinausea effect of ginger is well documented. From nausea resulting from chemotherapy and ocean travel to pregnancy and gynecological surgery,

ginger is the natural treatment of choice *(pg. 36)*.

18. Ginger, "the bioavailability herb," assists the digestion of other nutrients and is a recommended addition to natural supplement regimes *(pg. 40)*.

19. Parasites pose a much greater threat to the industrialized world than is generally recognized. Ginger exhibits a wide range of antiparasitic activities *(pg. 42)*.

20. The historic observation that ginger is a cold remedy is probably a result of a combination of principal actions including eicosanoid balance, probiotic support antitoxic and cytoprotective influences *(pg. 45)*.

21. Ginger possesses a significant antimutagenic potential against such powerful carcinogens as benzo(a)pyrene and the most toxic burnt byproducts of the amino acid tryptophan. Research also warrants further investigation into ginger's anticancer properties and its role in a cancer treatment program *(pg. 46)*.

22. Ginger has been shown to positively affect parameters of health such as cholesterol and blood sugar and balance numerous body systems including the circulatory, respiratory and reproductive systems. Ginger's beneficial effects have also been demonstrated in external treatments with dramatic results *(pg. 48)*.

23. Ginger is a remarkably safe herb. No modern pharmaceutical can compete with its range of therapeutic properties and absence of adverse side effects. Care and moderation should be exercised when using ginger during pregnancy and before surgery. Up to 2 grams daily of the powdered herb should be a safe preventive dosage for the general population. In all cases, introduction of ginger into the diet should be gradual *(pg. 50)*.

24. The effectiveness of ginger will be dependent upon the quality of the rhizome. Since commercial ginger is subject to many potential levels of chemical contamination, organically certified products are recommended *(pg. 54)*.

25. Both fresh and dry ginger are recommended forms for supplementation. There will be different properties gained from each. Ginger is commercially available as fresh, dried, and in syrup, capsules and extract *(pg. 54)*.

Freedom & Health at the Crossroads

26. With a health-care system that is widely recognized in crisis and in danger of bankrupting this country, natural and traditional remedies offer both a safe and economical potential to save lives and drastically improve the nation's health *(pg. 63)*.

27. Government and the pharmaceutical, food, medical and insurance industries have much at stake in the current system's continuity. Whether or not the public will ever realize the full daily tonic and healing value of ginger as well as the huge potential of countless other traditional remedies will be dependent upon the political strength of the growing "alternative" and self-health-care movements *(pg. 67)*.

Glossary•

ABORTIFACIENT	An agent that produces abortion.
ANALEPTIC	A restorative remedy; a central nervous system stimulant.
ANALGESIC	A condition in which stimuli are perceived but are not interpreted as pain; usually accompanied by sedation without loss of consciousness.
ANGINA PECTORIS	Severe constricting pain in the chest, often radiating from the pericardium to the left shoulder and down the arm, due to ischemia of the heart muscle usually caused by coronary disease.
ANTHELMINTIC	An agent that destroys or expels intestinal worms.
ANTIBACTERIAL	Destructive to or preventing the growth of bacteria.
ANTICATHARTIC	An agent that inhibits purging or evacuating of the bowels.
ANTIDIABETIC	Preventing or inhibiting the development of diabetes (any of several metabolic disorders marked by excessive discharge of urine and persistent thirst).
ANTIEMETIC	A remedy that tends to control nausea and vomiting.

• Stedman Medical Dictionary 25th Edition was used in the preparation of this glossary.

ANTIFUNGAL	Inhibiting the growth of fungi, any of numerous plants of the division or subkingdom Thallophyta, lacking chlorophyll and including yeasts, molds, smuts and mushrooms.
ANTI-INFLAMMATORY	Reducing inflammation by acting on body mechanisms, without directly antagonizing the causative agent; denoting agents such as antihistamines and glucocorticoids.
ANTIMETASTATIC	Preventing the shifting of a disease from one part of the body to another part.
ANTIMUTAGENIC	Inhibiting the ability to cause cell mutations and subsequently cancer.
ANTIOXIDANT	An agent that inhibits oxidation and thus prevents rancidity of oils or fats or the deterioration of other materials through oxidative processes.
ANTIPYRETIC	An agent that reduces fever.
ANTITHROMBIC	Inhibiting or preventing the effects of thrombin (an enzyme in blood that facilitates blood clotting) in such a manner that blood does not coagulate.
ANTITUMOR	Inhibiting the development of tumors or swellings in the body.
ANTITUSSIVE	A cough remedy or reliever.
ANTIULCER	Inhibiting the development of ulcers or lesions on the surface of the skin or a mucous surface, caused by superficial loss of tissue, usually from inflammation.

ANTIVIRAL	Inhibiting the development of a virus, any of various submicroscopic pathogens consisting essentially of a core of a single nucleic acid surrounded by a protein coat, having the ability to replicate only inside a living cell.
APHRODISIAC	Anything that arouses or increases sexual desire.
ARRHYTHMIA	Loss of rhythm, denoting especially irregularity of the heartbeat.
ARTERIOSCLEROSIS	Hardening of the arteries.
BIOAVAILABILITY	The physiological availability of a given amount of a drug, as distinct from its chemical potency.
CARDIOTONIC	Exerting a favorable effect upon the action of the heart.
CARMINATIVE	Preventing the formation or causing the expulsion of flatus; an agent that relieves flatulence.
COLITIS	Inflammation of the colon.
CYTOTOXIC	Detrimental or destructive to cells.
DIAPHORETIC	An agent that increases perspiration.
EICOSANOIDS	The physiologically active substances derived from arachidonic acid, i.e., the prostaglandins, leukotrienes, and thromboxanes. Also known as the arachidonic acid cascade.
EMMENAGOGUE	An agent that induces or increases menstrual flow.
ENZYME	Organic catalyst; a protein, secreted by cells, that acts as a catalyst to induce chemical changes in other substances, itself remaining apparently unchanged by the process.

EXPECTORANT	An agent promoting secretion from the mucous membrane of the air passages or facilitates its expulsion.
FEBRIFUGE	An agent that reduces fever.
FILARIASIS	The presence of filariae or nematodes in the tissues of the body, or in flood or tissue fluids.
FUMIGANT	Any vaporous substance used as a disinfectant or pesticide.
FUNGICIDE	Any substance that has a destructive killing action upon fungi.
GALACTAGOGUE	An agent that promotes the secretion and flow of milk.
HEPATOTOXIC	Relating to an agent that damages the liver, or pertaining to any such action.
HYPOCHOLESTEREMIC	Denoting the presence of abnormally small amounts of cholesterol in the circulating blood.
HYPOGLYCEMIA	An abnormally small concentration of glucose in the circulating blood, i.e., less than the minimum of the normal range.
IMMUNE SUPPORTIVE	Aiding in the resistance to an infectious disease; helping to free from the possibility of acquiring a given infectious disease.
ISCHEMIC	Relating to or affected by ischemia—the local anemia due to mechanical obstruction (mainly arterial narrowing) of the blood supply.
LEUKOTRIENES	Products of arachidonic acid metabolism with postulated physiologic activity such as mediators of inflammation and roles in allergic reactions; differ from the related prostaglandins and thromboxanes by not having a central ring.

MUCOLYTIC	Capable of dissolving, digesting, or liquefying mucus.
MUTAGENIC	Having the power to cause cell mutations and subsequently cancer.
MYELOPOIESIS	Formation of the tissue elements of bone marrow, or any of the types of blood cells derived from bone marrow, or both processes.
NEMATODE	A common name for any roundworm of the phylum Nematoda.
NECROTIZING	Causing the pathologic death of one or more cells.
NEUTROPHIL	A mature white blood cell in the granulocytic series, formed by myelopoietic tissue of the bone marrow and released into the circulating blood.
OSTEOARTHRITIS	Degenerative joint disease; arthritis characterized by erosion of articular cartilage, either primary or secondary to trauma or other conditions, which becomes soft, frayed, and thinned; pain and loss of function result.
PANACEA	A cure-all; a remedy claimed to be curative of all diseases.
PARTURITION	The act of giving birth; childbirth.
PATHOGEN	Any agent that causes diseases.
PHAGOCYTOSIS	The process of the immune system in which ingestion and digestion by cells of solid substances, e.g., other cells, bacteria, bits of necrosed tissue, foreign particles.
PLACEBO	An inert compound identical in appearance with material being tested in experimental research, which may or may not be known to the physician and/or patient, administered to distinguish between drug action and

	suggestive effect of the material under study.
PLATELET AGGREGATION	A crowded mass or cluster of blood platelets.
PRE-ECLAMPSIA	Development of hypertension with proteinuria or edema, or both, due to pregnancy or the influence of a recent pregnancy; it occurs after the 20th week of gestation, but may develop before this time.
PROBIOTIC SUPPORT	Fostering symbiosis, the association of two organisms that enhance the life processes of both. Often used to describe dietary supplements which encourage a healthy microbial environment.
PROSTAGLANDIN	Any of a class of physiologically active substances present in many tissues, with effects such as vasodilation, vasoconstriction, stimulation of intestinal or bronchial smooth muscle, uterine stimulation, and antagonism to hormones influencing lipid metabolism.
RUBEFACIENT	Causing a reddening of the skin.
SCHISTOSOMIASIS	A chronic and often debilitative infection with a species of Schistosoma, a genus of digenetic trematodes, including the blood flukes of man and domestic animals.
SCIATICA	Pain in the lower back and hip radiating down the back of the thigh into the leg, usually due to herniated lumbar disk.
SEROTONIN	A vasoconstrictor, liberated by the blood platelets, that inhibits gastric secretion and stimulates smooth muscle.

SIALOGOGUE	An agent promoting the flow of saliva.
SYNERGIST	A structure, agent, or physiologic process that aids the action of another.
SYNTHETASE	An enzyme catalyzing the synthesis—or composition—of a specific substance.
THERMOREGULATORY	Controlling temperature.
THROMBOXANES	A group of compounds, included in the eicosanoids, formally based on thromboxane, but with the terminal COOH group present; biochemically related to the prostaglandins and formed from them through a series of steps involving the formation of an endoperoxide by a cyclooxy- genase. Thromboxanes are so named from their influence on platelet aggregation and the formation of the oxygen-containing six-membered ring.
THROMBOSIS	Clotting within a blood vessel which may cause infarction—or sudden insufficiency of blood supply—of tissues supplied by the vessel.
TREMATODE	Common name for a fluke of the class Trematoda, flatworms with leaf-shaped bodies and two muscular suckers.
ULCEROGENIC	Ulcer-producing.
VASOCONSTRICTION	Narrowing of the blood vessels.
VASOSPASM	Contraction or hypertonia of the muscular coats of the blood vessels.

Ginger's Constituents & Actions

An herb is an infinitely complex array of elements. To create an observed therapeutic effect, each of these hundreds of elements interact with the others in a cascade which defies explanation. This section is included to give the reader a sense of just how miraculous a plant's activities are and how presumptious it is to think that one can isolate an "active" element from a plant.

Although there are serious limitations to active constituent isolation, this breakdown on ginger does reveal a daunting array of elements. Many of these compounds have collectively been the subject of literally thousands of studies. Of particular note are ascorbic acid, caffeic acid, capsaicin, beta-carotene, curcumin, lecithin, limonene, quercetin, selenium and tryptophan.

This section combines the monumental works of James Duke, USDA botanist, and Norman Farnsworth, Research Professor.[314-315]

ACETALDEHYDE: fungicide respiroparalytic

ACETIC-ACID: antiotitic, antivaginitic, bactericide, expectorant, fungicide, mucolytic, osteolytic, protisticide, spermicide, ulcerogenic, verrucolytic

ACETONE: CNS-depressant, narcotic

ALANINE: Cancer-preventive

ALBUMIN

ALLO-AROMADENDRENE

ALLO-AROMADENDRINE

ALUMINUM: Antivaginitic, candidicide, encephalopathic

GAMMA-AMINOBUTYRIC-ACID: analeptic, antihypertensive, antilethargic, diuretic, neurotransmitter

ANGELICOIDENOL-2-0-BETA-D-GLUCOPYRANOSIDE

ARGININE: antiencephalopathic, antihepatitic, anti-infertility?, diuretic

AROMADENDRENE

AROMADENDRIN: cancer-preventive

ASCORBIC-ACID: antiChron's, anticold, antidecubitic, antidote (paraquat), antiedemic, antilepric, antimigraine, antinitrosic, antioxidant, antiscorbutic, antiseptic, cancer-preventive, detoxicant, diuretic, hypotensive, mucolytic, urinary-acidulant, vulnerary

ASH

ASPARAGINE: antisickling, diuretic

ASPARTIC-ACID: anti-morphinic, neuroexcitant

BENZALDEHYDE: anesthetic, antipeptic, antiseptic, antispasmodic, antitumor, insectifuge, narcotic

3-PHENYL BENZALDEHYDE

4-PHENYL BENZALDEHYDE

BISABOLENE

BETA-BISABOLENE

BETA-BISABOLOL

BORNEOL: analgesic, anti-inflammatory, febrifuge, hepatoprotectant, berbicide, insectifuge, spasmolytic

D-BORNEOL

BORNEOL ACETATE

(+)-BORNEOL

ISO-BORNEOL

BORNYL-ACETATE: antifeedant, bactericide, insectifuge, viricide

BORON: androgenic, antiosteoporotic, estrogenic

SEC-BUTANOL

TERT-BUTANOL

N-BUTYRALDEHYDE

ALPHA-CADINENE

DELTA-CADINENE

ALPHA-CADINOL

CAFFEIC-ACID: antiflu, antihepatotoxic, antiherpetic, antioxidant, antiseptic, antispasmodic, antitumor, antitumor-promoter, antiviral, bactericide, cancer-preventive, choleretic, fungicide, hepatoprotective, hepatotropic, histamine-inhibitor, leukotriene-inhibitor, lipoxygenase-inhibitor, tumorigenic, viricide, vulnerary

CALAMENENE

CALCIUM

CAMPHENE: insectifuge

CAMPHENE-HYDRATE

CAMPHOR: allelopathic, analgesic, anesthetic, antifeedant, antifibrositic, antineuralgic, antipruritic, antiseptic, cancer-preventive, carminative, CNS-stimulant, convulsant, counterirritant, deliriant, ecbolic, emetic, expectorant, herbicide, insectifuge, respiroinhibitor, rubefacient, stimulant

CAPRIC-ACID: fungicide

CAPRYLIC-ACID: candidicide, fungicide

CAPSAICIN: analgesic, anesthetic, antiaggregant, anti-inflammatory, antineuralgic, antinociceptive, antioxidant, antiulcer, cancer-preventive, carcinogenic, cardiotonic, cyclooxygenase-inhibitor, diaphoretic, hypothermic, irritant, 5-lipoxygenase-inhibitor, neurotoxic, repellant, respirosensitizer, sialogogue

CARBOHYDRATES

CAR-3-ENE

DELTA-CAR-3-ENE: bactericide, anti-inflammatory, insectifuge

BETA-CAROTENE: antiacne, antiaging, anticoronary, antilupus, antiozenic, antiphotophobic, antiPMS, antiporphyric, antitumor, antiulcer, cancer-preventive, immunostimulant

CARYOPHYLLENE: antiedemic, anti-inflammatory, insectifuge, perfumery, spasmolytic, termitifuge

BETA-CARYOPHYLLENE

CEDOROL

CHAVICOL: fungicide, nematicide

CHLOROGENIC-ACID: allergenic, antifeedant, antihepatotoxic, antioxidant, antipolio, antiseptic, anti-tumor-promoter, antiviral, bactericide, cancer-preventive, choleretic, clastogenic, diuretic, histamine-inhibitor, juvabional, leukotriene-inhibitor, lipoxygenase-inhibitor

CHROMIUM: Insulinogenic

CINEOL

1,8-CINEOL: allelopathic, anesthetic, antibronchitic, anticatarrh, antilaryngitic, antipharyngitic, antirhinitic, antiseptic, antitussive, bactericide, choleretic, CNS-stimulant, counterirritant, dentifrice, expectorant, fungicide, hepatotonic, herbicide, hypotensive, insectifuge, rubefacient, sedative

2-HYDROXY-1,8-CINEOL

CITRAL: antihistaminic, antiseptic, bactericide, cancer-preventive, fungicide, herbicide, perfumery, sedative, teratogenic

CITRONELLAL: antiseptic, bactericide, embryotoxic, insectifuge, perfumery, sedative, tertogenic

CITRONELLOL: bactericide, candidicide, fungicide, herbicide, perfumery, sedative

CITRONELLYL-ACETATE

COBALT

ALPHA-COPAENE

COPPER: contraceptive

P-COUMARIC-ACID: antineoplastic, bactericide, cancer-preventive, choleretic, lipoxygenase-inhibitor, prostaglandin-synthesis-inhibitor

CUMENE: narcotic

ALPHA-CURCUMENE: antitumor, anti-inflammatory

(+)-ALPHA-CURCUMENE

AR-CURCUMEN

CURCUMIN: antiaggregant, anticholecystitic, antiedemic, anti-inflammatory, antilymphomic, antimutagenic, antiprostaglandin, antitumor, anti-tumor-promoter, bactericide, cancer-preventive, cardiodepressant, cholagogue, choleretic, cyclooxygenase-inhibitor, cytotoxic, dye, fungicide, hepatoprotective, hypotensive, 5-lipoxygenase-inhibitor, spasmolytic

DEMETHYL-HEXAHYDRO-CURCUMIN

P-CYMENE: analgesic, antiflu, antirheumatalgic, bactericide, fungicide, herbicide, insectifuge, viricide

P-CYMEN-8-OL

CYSTEINE: antiaddisonian, anticytotoxic, antiophthalmic, antioxidant, antitumor, antiulcer, cancer-preventive, detoxicant

CYSTINE: adjuvant, antihomocystinuric

DECANAL

N-DECANAL

3-6-EPOXY-1-(4-HYDROXY-3-METHOXY-PHENYL) DECA-3-5-DIENE

3(R)-5(S)-DIACETOXY-1-(3-4-DIMETHOXY-PHENYL) DECANE

3(R)-5(S)-DIACETOXY-1-(4-HYDROXY-3-METHOXY-PHENYL) DECANE

3(R)-ACETOXY-5(S)-HYDROXY-1-(4-HYDROXY-3-METHOXY-PHENYL) DECANE

5(S)-3(R)-DIHYDROXY-1-(4-HYDROXY-3-METHOXY-PHENYL) DECANE

5(S)-ACETOXY-3(R)-HYDROXY-1-(4-HYDROXY-3-METHOXY-PHENYL) DECANE

DECYLALDEHYDE

6-DEHYDROGINGERDIONE: prostaglandin-suppressor

6,10-DEHYDROGINGERDIONE

10-DEHYDROGINGERDIONE: anticholeretic, prostaglandin-suppressor

6-DIHYDROGINGERDIONE

DELPHINIDIN: allelochemic, cancer-preventive

DIETHYLSULFIDE

DODECANOIC-ACID

BETA-ELEMENE

ELEMOL

ESSENTIAL OIL

10-EPIZONARENE

8-BETA-17-EPOXY-LABD-TRANS-12-ENE-15,16-DIAL

ETHYL-ACETATE: antispasmodic, carminative, CNS-depressant, stimulant

ETHYL-ISOPROPYL-SULFIDE

ETHYL-MYRISTATE

BETA-EUDESMOL: antianoxic, antipeptic, CNS-inhibitor, hepatoprotective

GAMMA-EUDESMOL

METHYL-ETHER-ISO-EUGENOL

FARNESAL: juvabional

FARNESENE

ALPHA-FARNESENE

TRANS-ALPHA-FARNESENE

BETA-FARNESENE

TRANS-BETA-FARNESENE: pheromone

FARNESOL: juvabional, perfumery

FAT

FERULIC-ACID: allelopathic, analgesic, antiaggregant, antidysmenorrheic, antispasmodic, antitumor, anti-tumor-promoter, antiviral, arteriodilator, bactericide, cancer-preventive, cardiac, choleretic, fungicide, hepatotropic, preservative, uterosedative

FIBER: antitumor, antidiabetic, antiobesity, cancer-preventive, cardioprotective, hypocholesteremic, hypotensive,laxative

FLUORIDE

FLUORINE

FRUCTOSE: antiketotic, neoplastic

FURANOGERMENONE

FURFURAL: antiseptic, fungicide, insecticide

GALANOLACTONE

GADOLEIC-ACID

GERANIAL: bactericide

CIS-GERANIC-ACID

TRANS-GERANIC-ACID

GERANIOL: antiseptic, cancer-preventive, candidicide, embryotoxic, fungicide, insectifuge, insectiphile, perfumery, sedative

GERANIOL ACETATE

GERANYL-ACETATE

GERMANIUM

GINGEDIACETATE

6-GINGEDIOL

6-GINGEDIOL-ACETATE

6-GINGEDIOL-ACETATE-METHYL-ETHER

6-GINGEDIOL-DIACETATE

6-GINGEDIOL-DIACETATE-METHYL-ETHER

6-GINGEDIOL-METHYL-ETHER

8-GINGEDIOL

10-GINGEDIOL

6-GINGERDIONE: prostaglandin-suppressor

10-GINGERDIONE: prostaglandin-suppressor

6-10-GINGERDIONE

GINGERENONE-A: anticoccidioid, fungicide

GINGERENONE-B: fungicide

GINGERENONE-C: fungicide

GINGERGLYCOLIPID-A

GINGERGLYCOLIPID-B

GINGERGLYCOLIPID-C

GINGEROL: cancer-preventive, hepatoprotective, molluscicide

4-GINGEROL

6-GINGEROL: analgesic, anti-5-HT, antiemetic, antipyretic, antitussive, cardiotonic, cholagogue, depressor, hepatoprotective, hypotensive, prostaglandin-suppressor, sedative

(+)-6-GINGEROL

(S)(+)-6-GINGEROL

6-GINGEROL-METHYL

7-GINGEROL

8-GINGEROL: anti-5-HT, cardiotonic, enteromotility-enhancer

8-GINGEROL-METHYL

9-GINGEROL

10-GINGEROL: cardiotonic

10-GINGEROL-METHYL

12-GINGEROL

12-GINGEROL-METHYL

14-GINGEROL

16-GINGEROL

DIHYDRO-GINGEROL

GINGEROL-METHYL

GINGEROL-METHYL-ETHER

GINGERONE

6-GINGESULFONIC ACID

GLANOLACTONE

GLANOLACTONE GLOBULIN

GLUCOSE: acetylcholinergic, antihepatotoxic, antiketotic, hyperglycemic, memory-enhancer

GLUTAMIC-ACID: antalkali?, antiepileptic, antihyperammonemic, antiretardation, anxiolytic

GLUTELIN

GLYCINE: antiacid, antidote, antiencephalopathic, antigastritic, antipruritic, antiulcer, cancer-preventive

GLYOXAL

GUAIOL: termitifuge

6-METHYL-HEPT-5-EN-2-OL

6-METHYL-HEPT-5-EN-2-ONE

HEPTAN-2-OL

HEPTAN-2-ONE

2-2-4-TRIMETHYL-HEPTANE

3(S)-5(S)-DIACETOXY-1-(4'-HYDROXY-3'-5'-DIMETHOXY-PHENYL)-7-(4"-HYDROXY-3"-METHOXY-PHENYL HEPTANE

3(S)-5(S)-DIHYDROXY-1-(4'-hYDROXY-3'-5'-DIMETHOXY-PHENYL)-7-(4"-HYDROXY-3"-METHOXY-PHENYL) HEPTANE

3-5-DIACETOXY-1-(4-HYDROXY-3-5-DIMETHOXY-PHENYL)-7-(4-HYDROXY-3-METHOXY-PHENYL) HEPTANE

3-5-DIACETOXY-1-7-BIS-(4-HYDROXY-3-METHOXY-PHENYL) MESO-HEPTANE

N-HEPTANE

1-7-BIS-(4-HYDROXY-3-METHOXY-PHENYL) HEPTANE-3(S)-DIOL

METHYL-HEPTENONE

HEXAHYDROCURCUMIN: choleretic, cholagogue

HEXAN-1-AL

HEXAN-1-OL

HEXANOL: antiseptic

CIS-HEXAN-3-OL

BETA-HIMACHALENE: anti-inflammatory, insecticide

HISTIDINE: antiarteriosclerotic, antiulcer

HUMULENE

P-HYDROXYBENZOIC-ACID: antisickling, bactericide, cancer-preventive

1-(4-HYDROXY-3-METHOXYPHENYL)-3,5-OCTANEDIOL

1-(4-HYDROXY-3-METHOXYPHENYL)-3,5-DIACETOXYOCTANE

BETA-IONONE: cancer-preventive

IRON: antiakathisic, antienemic

ISOEUGENOL-METHYL-ETHER

ISOGINGERENONE-B: fungicide

ISOLEUCINE: antiencephalopathic?, antipellagric

ISOVALERALDEHYDE

JUNIPER CAMPHOR

KAEMPFEROL: antifertility, antihistaminic, anti-inflammatory, antioxidant, antispasmodic, anti-tumor-promoter, anti-ulcer, cancer-preventive, choleretic, diuretic, HIV-RT-inhibitor, hypotensive, mutagenic, natriuretic, spasmolytic, teratologic

KILOCALORIES

LAURIC-ACID

LECITHIN: antialzheimeran, antiataxic, anticirrhotic, antidementic, antidyskinetic, antieczemic, antimorphinistic, antioxidant (synergist), antipsoriac, anti-sclerodermic, antiseborrheic, antisprue, antiTourette's, cholinogenic, hepatoprotective, hypocholesterolemic, lipotropic

LEUCINE: antiencephalopathic

ISO-LEUCINE

LIMONENE: achE-inhibitor, anticancer, antilithic, bactericide, cancer-preventive, herbicide, insectifuge, insecticide, irritant, sedative, viricide

LINALOOL: antiseptic, bactericide, cancer-preventive, fungicide, insectifuge, perfumery, sedative, spasmolytic, termitifuge, tumor-promoter, viricide

LINALOOL OXIDE

TRANS-LINALOOL-OXIDE

LINOLEIC-ACID: antiarteriosclerotic, antifibrinolytic, antigranular, cancer-preventive, hepatoprotective, insectifuge

ALPHA-LINOLENIC-ACID: cancer-preventive

LYSINE: antialkalotic, hypoarginanemic

MAGNESIUM: hypotensive

MANGANESE: antianemic, antidyskinetic

P-MENTHA-1-5-DIEN-7-OL

P-MENTHA-2-8-DIEN-1-OL

P-MENTHAL-1-5-DIEN-8-OL

MENTHOL-ACETATE

P-METHA-1-8-DIEN-7-OL

METHIONINE: antidote (acetominaphen, paracetamol), antieczemic, cancer-preventive, emetic, glutathionigenic, hepatoprotective, lipotropic, urine-acidifier, urine-deodorant

METHYL-ACETATE

METHYL-CAPRYLATE

6-METHYLGINGEDIACETATE

6-METHYLGINGEDIOL

METHYL-GLYOXAL

METHYL-ISOBUTYL-KETONE

METHYL-NONYL-KETONE

METHYL-6-SHOGAOL

METHYL-8-SHOGAOL

METHYL-10-SHOGAOL

MUFA

ALPHA-MUUROLENE

GAMMA-MUUROLENE

MYRCENE: antinociceptive, bactericide, insectifuge, spasmolytic

BETA-MYRCENE: cancer-preventive, perfumery

MYRICETIN: allelochemic, antifeedant, antigastric, anti-inflammatory, cancer-preventive, diuretic, larvistat

MYRISTIC-ACID: cancer-preventive, cosmetic

MYRTENAL

NEOISOPULEGOL

NERAL: bactericide

NEROL: bactericide, perfumery

NEROL OXIDE

NEROLIDOL

9-OXO-NEROLIDOL

TRANS-NEROLIDOL

NIACIN: antiacrodynic, antiamplyopic, antianginal, antidysphagic, antineuralgic, antipellagric, antiscotomic, antivertigo, cancer-preventive, hepatoprotective, hypoglycemic, vasodilator

NICKEL

NITROGEN

NONANAL

N-NONANE

N-NONANONE

NONYL-ALDEHYDE

NONAN-2-OL

N-NONANOL

NONAN-2-ONE

2-6-DIMETHYL OCTA-2-6-DIENE-1-8-DIOL

2-6-DIMETHYL OCTA-3-7-DIENE-1-6-DIOL

OCTAN-1-AL

OCTAN-2-OL

N-OCTANE

N-OCTANOL

TRANS-OCTEN-2-AL

OLEIC-ACID: anemiagenic, cancer-preventive, choleretic, insectifuge, irritant, percutaneostimulant

OXALIC-ACID: antiseptic, fatal?, hemostatic, renotoxic

9-OXO-NEROLIDOL

PALMITIC-ACID: antifibrinolytic

PALMITOLEIC-ACID

PANTOTHENIC-ACID

PARADOL

6-PARADOL

PATCHOULI-ALCOHOL: antiplaque, bactericide, fungicide

PENTAN-2-OL

PENTOSANS

PERILLEN

PERILLENE

ALPHA-PHELLANDRENE: insectiphile

BETA-PHELLANDRENE: perfumery

(+)-BETA-PHELLANDRENE

PHENYLALANINE: anti-attention-deficit-disorder, antidepressant, antiparkinsonian, antisickling, antivitiligic, tremorigenic

PHOSPHATIDIC-ACID

PHOSPHORUS

PHYTOSTEROLS

ALPHA-PINENE: allelochemic, anti-inflammatory, cancer-preventive, coleoptiphile, insectfuge, insectiphile

BETA-PINENE: insectifuge

PIPECOLIC-ACID

POTASSIUM

PROLAMINE

PROLINE

N-PROPANOL

PROPIONALDEHYDE

PROTEIN

NEO-ISO-PULEGOLE

PUFA : antiacne, antieczemic, antiMS, antipolyneuritic

QUERCETIN: aldose-reductase-inhibitor, allelochemic, antiaggregant, antiallergenic, antianaphylactic, anticataract, antidermatitic, antifeedant, antiflu, antigastric, antihepatotoxic, antiherpetic, antihistaminic, antihydrophobic, anti-inflammatory, antileukotrienic, anti-lipoperoxidant, antioxidant, antipermeability, antiradicular, antispasmodic, antitumor, antiviral, bactericide, cancer-preventive, capillariprotective, cytotoxic, HIV-RT-inhibitor, juvabional, larvistat, lipoxygenase-inhibitor, mast-cell-stabilizer, mutagenic, spasmolytic, teratologic, tumorigenic, vasodilator, xanthine-oxidase-inhibitor

RAFFINOSE

RIBOFLAVIN: antiarabiflavinotic, anticheilotic, antidecubitic, antikeratitic, antimigraine, antipellagric, antiphotophobic, cancer-preventive

ROSEFURAN

SABINENE

CIS-SELINEN-4-OL

ALPHA-SELINENE

BETA-SELINENE

GAMMA-SELINENE

SELENIUM: anorexic, antidote (mercury), antikeshan, antiosteoarthritic, antioxidant, antiulcerogenic, cancer-preventive, depressant, prostaglandin-sparer

SELINA-3-7(11)-DIENE

SERINE: cancer-preventive

CIS-SESQUIABINENE-HYDRATE

SESQUIPHELLANDRENE

BETA-SESQUIPHELLANDRENE

BETA-SESQUIPHELLANDROL

CIS-BETA-SESQUIPHELLANDROL

TRANS-BETA-SESQUIPHELLANDROL

CIS-SESQUISABINENE-HYDRATE

SESQUITERPENE ALCOHOL

SESQUITERPENE HYDROCARBON

SESQUITHUJENE

SFA

SHIKIMIC-ACID: bruchifuge, carcinogenic, ileorelaxant, mutagenic

SHOGAOL: anti-inflammatory, cyclooxygenase-inhibitor, hypotensive, 5-lipoxygenase-inhibitor, molluscicide

6-SHOGAOL: analgesic, anti-5-HT, antipyretic, antitussive, CNS-depressant, en- teromotility-enhancer, hepatoprotective, hypotensive, prostaglandin-suppressor, sedative, sympathomimetic, vasoconstrictor

CIS-6-SHOGAOL

ANTI-METHYL-6-SHOGAOL

SYN-METHYL-6-SHOGAOL

TRAN-6-SHOGOAL

8-SHOGAOL

CIS-8-SHOGAOL

ANTI-METHYL-8-SHOGAOL

SYN-METHYL-8-SHOGAOL

TRAN-8-SHOGAOL

10-SHOGAOL

CIS-10-SHOGAOL

ANTI-METHYL-10-SHOGAOL

SYN-METHYL-10-SHOGAOL

TRANS-10-SHOGAOL

CIS-12-SHOGAOL

TRANS-12-SHOGAOL

SILICON

BETA-SITOSTEROL: androgenic, anorexic, antiadenomic, antiandrogenic, antiestrogenic, antifeedant, antifertility, antigonadotrophic, anti-inflammatory, antileukemic, antimutagenic, antiprogestational, antiprostatadenomic, antiprostatitic, antitumor, artemicide, bactericide, cancer-preventive, candidicide, estrogenic, gonadotrophic, hypocholesterolemic, hypolipidemic, spermicide, viricide

SODIUM

STARCH: absorbent, antinesidioblastosic, emollient, poultice

STEARIC-ACID

SUCROSE

ETHYL-ISO-PROPYL-SULFIDE

METHYL-ALLYL-SULFIDE

1-8-TERPINE HYDRATE

TERPINEN-4-OL: antiallergic, antiasthmatic, antiseptic, antitussive, bacteriostatic, fungicide, herbicide, insectifuge, spermicide

ALPHA-TERPINENE: insectifuge

GAMMA-TERPINENE: insectifuge

4-TERPINEOL

ALPHA-TERPINEOL: termiticide

TERPINOLENE

THIAMIN: antialcoholic, antiberiberi, antocardiospasmic, anticolitic, antidecubitic, antideliriant, antiencephalopathic, antiheartburn, antiherpetic, antimigraine, antimyocarditic, antineaurasthenic, antineuritic, antipoliomyelitic, insectifuge

THREONINE: antiulcer

BETA-THUJONE: insectifuge

TIN: antiacne, bactericide, taenicide

TRICYCLENE

2,2,4-TRIMETHYL-HEPTANE

TRYPTOPHAN: analgesic, antidepressant, antidyskinetic, antihypertensive, antimigraine, antiphenylketonutic, antipsychotic, antirheumatic, carcinogenic, hypnotic, insulinotonic, sedative, serotonigenic, tumor-promoter

TYROSINE: antidepressant?, antiencephalopathic, antiphenylketonuric, cancer-preventive

UNDECAN-2-OL

N-UNDECANONE

UNDECAN-2-ONE

VALERALDEHYDE

VALINE: antiencephalopathic

VANILLIC-ACID: antifatigue, anthelmintic, antioxidant, antisickling, ascaricide, bactericide, cancer-preventive, choleretic, laxative

VANILLIN: allelochemic, cancer-preventive, fungicide, insectifuge?

VIT-B6

WATER

XANTHORRHIZOL

ALPHA-YLANGENE

ZINGERONE: anti-inflammatory, cyclo- oxygenase-inhibitor, hypotensive, 5-lipoxygenase-inhibitor, paralytic, vasodilator

ZINGIBAIN: proteolytic

ZINC: antiacne?, antiacrodermatitic, antianorexic, antiarthritic?, anticoeliac, anticold, antidote (cadmium), antiencephalopathic, antifuruncular, antiherpetic?, antiimpotence, antilepric, antiplaque, antistomatitic, antiulcer, antiulcer, antiviral?, astringent, deordorant, immunosuppressant, mucogenic, trichomonicide, vulnerary

ALPHA-ZINGIBENENE

ZINGIBERENE: antiulcer

ZINGIBERENE

ALPHA-ZINGIBERENE

BETA-ZINGIBERENE

ZINGIBERENOL

ZINGIBERINE

ZINGIBEROL

ZINGIBERONE

ZONARENE

ZT: hypocholesteremic

References

1. Govindarajan, V.S. "Ginger—Chemistry, technology, and quality evaluation: part 1." CRITICAL REVIEWS IN FOOD SCIENCE AND NUTRITION 1982;17(1):1-96 (p.1), citing Parry, J., *Spices*. Vols. 1 & 2, Chemical Publ. Co., New York, 1969.

2. Ibid., p. 29.

2a. McCaleb, R.S. "Rational Regulation of Herbal Products, Testimony before the Subcommittee on Government Operations." Herb Research Foundation, Washington, D.C., July 20, 1993.

2b. Eisenberg, D.M., Kessler, R.C., Foster, C., Norlock, F.E., Calkins, D.R., Delbanco, T.L. "Unconventional medicine in the United States. Prevalence, costs, and patterns of use." NEW ENGLAND JOURNAL OF MEDICINE 1993, Jan 28;328(4):246-52.

3. *Eating Well*, March-April 1993, p. 51.

4. Govindarajan, V.S. "Ginger—Chemistry, technology, and quality evaluation: part 1." CRITICAL REVIEWS IN FOOD SCIENCE AND NUTRITION 1982;17(1):1-96 (p.1), citing Parry, J., *Spices*. Vols. 1 and 2, Chemical Publ. Co., New York, 1969, p. 2-5.

5. Lawrence, B. "Major Tropical Spices — Ginger (Zingiber officinale Rosc.)." PERFUMER AND FLAVORIST Vol. 9, Oct/Nov 1984 2-38 (p. 3).

6. Govindarajan, V.S. "Ginger—Chemistry, technology, and quality evaluation: part 1." CRITICAL REVIEWS IN FOOD SCIENCE AND NUTRITION 1982;17(1):1-96 (p. 2-5).

7. Lad, V., Frawley, D. *Yoga of Herbs*, Lotus Press, Santa Fe, N.M.,1986, p. 122

8. Atal, C.K., Zutshi, U., Rao, P.G. "Scientific evidence on the role of Ayurvedic herbals on bioavailability of drugs." JOURNAL OF ETHNOPHARMACOLOGY 1981 Sep;4(2):229-32.

9. Sakai, Y., et al. "Effects of medicinal plant extracts from Chinese herbal medicines on the mutagenic activity of benzo(a)pyrene." MUTATION RESEARCH 206 (1988) 327-334.

10. Lawrence, B., "Major Tropical Spices — Ginger (Zingiber officinale Rosc.)." PERFUMER AND FLAVORIST Vol. 9, Oct/Nov 1984 2-38 (p.2).

11. Govindarajan, V.S. "Ginger—Chemistry, technology, and quality evaluation: part 1." CRITICAL REVIEWS IN FOOD SCIENCE AND NUTRITION 1982;17(1):1-96 (p.1).

12. Krochmal, C. "Ginger-Nutritional Value of Herbs." *Herb News* Spring 1981, p. 24.

13. Ody, P. *The Complete Medicinal Herbal*. Dorling Kindersley, London, 1993.

14. Felter, H.W., Lloyd, J.U. *King's American Dispensatory*. Eclectic Medical, 1983, p. 2111.

15. Kuts-Cheraux, A.W. *Naturae Medicina & Naturopathic Dispensatory*. Antioch Press, Yellow Springs, Ohio, 1953, p. 279.

16. Ellingwood, F., Lloyd, J.U. *American Materia Medica Therapeutics and Pharmacognosy*. Evanston, Ill. pp. 279-80.

17. Holdsworth, D., Wamoi, B. "Medicinal plants of the Admiralty Islands, Papua New Guinea. Part I." INT J CRUDE DRUG RES 1982;20(4):169-181.

18. Van Den Berg, M.A. "Ver-O-Peso: The ethnobotany of an Amazonian market." In G.T. Prance & J.A. Kallunki (eds), *Advances in Economic Botany Ethnobotany in the Neotropics*. N.Y. Botanical Garden, Bronx, N.Y., 1984, pp. 140-149.

19. Lucas, R. *Secrets of the Chinese Herbalists*. Parker Publishing Co., New York, 1977.

20. Kiuchi, F., Shibuya, M., Sankawa, U. "Inhibitors of prostaglandin biosynthesis from ginger." CHEMICAL AND PHARMACEUTICAL BULLETIN (Tokyo) 1982 Feb;30(2):754-7.

21. Yamahara, J., Miki, K., Chisaka, T., Sawada, T., Fujimura, H., Tomimatsu, T., Nakano, K., Nohara, T. "Cholagogic effect of ginger and its active constituents." JOURNAL OF ETHNOPHARMACOLOGY 1985 May;13(2):217-25.

22. Roig, Y., Mesa, J.T. *Plantas Medicinales, Aromaticas o Venenosas de Cuba*. Ministerio de Agricultura, Republica de Cuba, Havana, 1945, 872 pp.

23. Liu, W.H.D. "Ginger root, a new

antiemetic." ANAESTHESIA (U.K.) 1991; 45(12):1085ff.

24. Singh, Y.N. "Traditional medicine in Fiji: Some herbal folk cures used by Fiji Indians." J ETHNOPHARMACOL 1986;15(1):57-88.

25. Jain, S.K., Tarafder, C.R. "Medicinal plant-lore of the Santals." ECON BOT 1970;24:241-278.

26. Puri, H.S., Pandey, G. "Glimpses into the crude drugs of Sikkim." BULL MED ETHNOBOT RES 1980;1:55-71.

27. Reddy, M.B., Rebby, K.R., Reddy, M.N. "A survey of plant crude drugs of Anantapur District, Andhra Pradesh, India." INT J CRUDE DRUG RES 1989;27(3):145-155.

28. Comley, J.C.W. "New macrofilaricidal leads from plants?" TROP MED PARASITOL 1990;41(1):1-9.

29. Rao, R.R., Jamir, N.S. "Ethnobotanical studies in Nagaland. I. Medicinal plants." ECON BOT 1982;36:176-181.

30. John, D. "One hundred useful raw drugs of the Kani tribes of Trivandrum Forest Division, Kerala, India." INT J CRUDE DRUG RES 1984;22(1):17-39.

31. Alam, M., et al. "Treatment of diabetes through herbal drugs in rural India." FITOTHERAPIA 61:3, 1990, p. 240-2.

32. Mustafa, T., Srivastava, K.C. "Ginger (Zingiber officinale) in migraine headache." JOURNAL OF ETHNOPHARMACOLOGY 1990 Jul;29(3):267-73.

33. Tanaka, S., Saito, M., Tabata, M. "Bioassay of crude drugs for hair growth promoting activity in mice by a new simple method." PLANTA MED SUPPL 1980;40:84-90.

34. Hirschhorn, H.H. "Botanical remedies of the former Dutch East Indies (Indonesia). I. Eumycetes, pteridophyta, gymnospermae, angiosperme (monoctylendones only)." J ETHNOPHARMACOL 1983;7(2):123-156.

35. Burkill, I.H. *Dictionary of the Economic Products of the Malay Peninsula (Volume II).* Ministry of Agriculture & Cooperatives, Kuala Lumpur, Malaysia, 1966.

36. Sussman, L.K. "Herbal Medicine on Mauritius." J ETHNOPHARMACOL 1980;2:259-278.

37. Ishikura, N. "Flavonol glycosides in the flowers of hibiscus mutabilis f. versicolor." AGR BIOL CHEM 1982;46:1705-1706.

38. Sofowora, A. "The present status of knowledge of the plants used in traditional medicine in Western Africa: A medical approach and a chemical evaluation." J ETHNOPHARMACOL 1980;2:109-118.

39. Adewunmi, C.O., Oguntimein, B.O., Furu, P. "Molluscicidal and antischistosomal activities of Zingiber officinale." PLANTA MEDICA 1990 Aug;56(4):374-6.

40. Holdsworth, D., Pilokos, B., Lambes, P. "Traditional medicinal plants of New Ireland, Papua New Guinea." INT J CRUDE DRUG RES 1983;21(4):161-168.

41. Holdsworth, D., Rali, T. "A survey of medicinal plants of the Southern Highlands, Papua New Guinea." INT J CRUDE DRUG RES 1989;27(1):1-8.

42. Holdsworth, D. "Phytomedicine of the Madang Province, Papua New Guinea. Part I. Karkar Island." INT J CRUDE DRUG RES 1984;22(3):111-119.

43. Ramirez, V.R., Mostacero, L.J., Garcia, A.E., Majia, C.F., Pelaez, P.F., Medina, C.D., Miranda, C.H. *Vegetales Empleados en Medicina Tradcional Norperuana.* Banco Agario del Peru & Nacl Univ Trujillo, Trujillo, Peru, June 1988, 54pp.

44. Gonzalez, F., Silva, M. "A survey of plants with antifertility properties described in the South American folk medicine." Abstr Princess Congress I Bangkok Thailand, 10-13 December 1987, 20pp.

45. Velazco, E.A. "Herbal and traditional practices related to maternal and child health-care." RURAL RECONSTRUCTION REVIEW 1980:35-39.

46. Al-Yahya, M.A. "Phytochemical studies of the plants used in traditional medicine of Saudi Arabia." FITOTERAPIA 1986;57(3): 179-182.

47. Al-Yahya, M.A., Rafatullah, S., Mossa, J.S., Ageel, A.M., Parmar, N.S., Tariq, M. "Gastroprotective activity of ginger zingiber officinale rosc., in albino rats." AMER J CHIN MED 1989;17(1/2):51-56.

48. Woo, W.S., Lee, E.B., Shin, K.H., Kang, S.S., Chi, H.J. "A review of research on plants for fertility regulation in Korea." KOREAN J PHARMACOG 1981;12(3):153-170.

49. Hussein Ayoub, S.M., Baerheim-Suendsen, A. "Medicinal and aromatic plants in the Sudan: Usage and exploration." FITOTERAPIA 1981;52:243-246.

50. Haerdi, F. *Native medicinal plants of*

Ulanga District of Tanganyika (East Africa). Dissertation, Verlag fur Recht und Gesellschaft AG, Basel. Ph.D. Dissertation, Univ Basel 1964.

51. Watt, J.M., Breyer-Brandwijk, M.G. *The Medicinal and Poisonous Plants of Southern and Eastern Africa* (2d ed). E&S Livingstone Ltd., London, 1962.

52. Panthong, A., Tejasen, P. "Study of the effects and the mechanism of action of ginger (zingiber officinale roscoe) on motility of the intact intestine in dogs." CHIENG MAI MED BILL 1975;14(3):221-231.

53. Hantrakul, M., Tejason, P. "Study of the acute toxicity and cardiovascular effects of ginger (zingiber officinale roscoe)." THAI J PHARM SCI 1976;1(6):517-530.

54. Loewsoponkul, P. *Effect of Thai Emmenagogue Drugs on Rat Uterine.* Master's Thesis, Univ Bangkok, 1982, 96 pp.

55. Wasuwat, S. *A List of Thai Medicinal Plants, ASRCT, Bangkok.* ASRCT Research Report No. 1 on Res. Project. 17, 1967, 22 pp.

56. Ketusinh, O., Wimolwattanpun, S., Nilvises, N. "Smooth muscle actions of some Thai herbal carminatives." THAI J PHARMACOL 1984;6(1):11-19.

57. Panthong, A., Sivamogstham, P. "Pharmacological study of the action of ginger (zingiber officinale roscoe) on the gastrointestinal tract." CHIENG MAI MED BULL 1974;13(1):41-53.

58. *The Herbalist.* Hammond Book Company, Hammond, Indiana, 1931, 400 pp.

59. Grieve, M. Mrs. *A Modern Herbal (Vol. I).* Dover Publications, New York, 1971, p. 353-4.

60. Morton J.F. "Current folk remedies of northern Venezuela." Q J CRUDE DRUG RES 1975;13:97-121.

61. Petelot, A. *Les Plantes Medicinales du Cambodge, du Laos et du Vietnam* (Vols 1-4). Archives des Recherches Agronomiques et Pastorales au Vietnam, No. 23, 1954.

62. Fleurentin, J., Pelt, J.M. "Repertory of drugs and medicinal plants of Yemen." J ETHNOPHARMACOL 1982;6(1):85-108.

63. Felter, H.W., Lloyd, J.U. *King's American Dispensatory.* Eclectic Medical, 1983, pg. 2110.

64. *Napralert Constituent Report.*

65. Harborne, J., Baxter, H. *Phytochemistry Dictionary: A Handbook of Bioactive Compounds from Plants.* Taylor & Francis, Washington, D.C., 1993, p. 481.

66. *Phytochemical Dictionary,* J.B. Harborne, H. Baxter (eds), Taylor & Francis, Washington, D.C., 1993, p. 481.

67. Govindarajan, V.S. "Ginger-Chemistry, technology, and quality evaluation: part 2." CRITICAL REVIEWS IN FOOD SCIENCE AND NUTRITION 1982;17(3):189-258 (p. 230), citing Thompson, E.H., et al. "Ginger Rhizome: A new source of proteolytic enzyme." JOURNAL OF FOOD SCIENCE 38(4), 652-655, 1973.

68. Mowrey, D.B. *The Scientific Validation Of Herbal Medicine.* Cormorant Books, p. 261, citing Thompson, E.H., et al. "Ginger Rhizome: a new source of proteolytic enzyme." JOURNAL OF FOOD SCIENCE 38(4), 652-655, 1973.

69. Lawrence, B. "Major Tropical Spices — Ginger (Zingiber officinale Rosc.)" PERFUMER AND FLAVORIST. Vol. 9, Oct/Nov 1984 2-38, citing Thompson, E.H., et al. "Ginger Rhizome: a new source of proteolytic enzyme." JOURNAL OF FOOD SCIENCE 38(4), 652-655, 1973.

70. Govindarajan, V.S. "Ginger-Chemistry, technology, and quality evaluation: part 2." CRITICAL REVIEWS IN FOOD SCIENCE AND NUTRITION 1982;17(3):189-258 (p. 230), citing Huhtanen, C. "Inhibition of Clostridium botulinum by spice extracts and aliphatic alcohols." J FOOD PROTECTION 43(3):195, 1980.

71. Gugnani, H.C., Ezenwanze, E.C. "Antibacterial activity of extracts of ginger and African oil bean seed." JOURNAL OF COMMUNICABLE DISEASES 1985 Sep;17(3):233-6.

72. Mascolo, N., Jain, R., Jain, S.C., Capasso, F. "Ethnopharmacologic investigation of ginger (Zingiber officinale)." JOURNAL OF ETHNOPHARMACOLOGY 1989 Nov;27(1-2):129-40.

73. Goto, C., Kasuya, S., Koga, K., Ohtomo, H., Kagei, N. "Lethal efficacy of extract from Zingiber officinale (traditional Chinese medicine) or [6]-shogaol and [6]-gingerol in Anisakis larvae in vitro." PARASITOLOGY RESEARCH 1990;76(8):653-6.

74. Raj, R. "Screening of some indigenous plants for anthelmintic action against human ascaris lumbricoides." INDIAN JOURNAL PHYSIOLOGY AND PHARMACOLOGY

18)2): 129-131, 1974.

75. Datta, A., Sukal, N. "Antifilarial effects of Zingiber officinale on Dirofilaria immitis." J. HELMINTHOL 61 (1987):268-270.

76. Kiuchi, F. "Nematocidal Activity Of Some Anthelmintics, traditional medicines, and spices by new assay method using larvae of toxocara canis." SHOYAKUGAKU ZASSHI 1989 43(4), 279-287.

77. Ibid., citing Kucera, M. (1975) NIGERIAN J PHARM 6,77.

78. Ibid., citing Kucera, M., Kucerova, H. J CHROMATOGRAPHY (1975) 93, 421.

79. Ibid., citing Kucera, M., Theakston, R., Kucerova, H. NIG J PHARM (1975)6, 121.

80. Ibid., citing Adewunmi, C., Sofowora, E.A. PLANTA MEDICA (1980)39,57.

81. Ibid., citing Sukul, N., et al. "Nematicidal action of some edible crops." NEMATOLOGICA 20, 187-191.

82. Rodeheaver, G., Marsh, D., Edgerton, M.T., Edlich, R.F. "Proteolytic enzymes as adjuncts to antimicrobial prophylaxis of contaminated wounds." AMERICAN JOURNAL OF SURGERY 1975 May;129(5):537-44.

83. Baskanchiladze, G.Sh., Khurtsilava, L.A., Gelovani, I.A., Asatiani, M.V., Rossinskii, V.I. "In combination with papain in experimental septicemia." ANTIBIOTIKI 1984 Jan;29(1):33-5.

84. Brisou, J., Babin, P., Babin, R. ["Potentialization of antibiotics by lytic enzymes"] COMPTES ["Chemotherapeutic effectiveness of antibiotics"] RENDUS DES SEANCES DE LA SOCIETE DE BIOLOGIE ET DE SES 1975;169(3):660-4.

85. Udod, V.M., Kolos, A.I., Gritsuliak, Z.N. ["Treatment of patients with lung abscess by local administration of papain"] VESTNIK KHIRURGII IMENI I. I. GREKOVA 1989 Mar;142(3):24-7.

86. Emeruwa, A.C. "Antibacterial substance from Carica papaya fruit extract." JOURNAL OF NATURAL PRODUCTS 1982 Mar-Apr;45(2):123-7.

87. Neubauer, R. "A plant protease for potentiation of and possible replacement of antibiotics." EXP MED SURG 19, 143-160, 1961.

88. Vogel, H. *The Nature Doctor.* Keats Publishing, New Canaan, Conn., 1991, p. 446.

89. Srivastava, K.C., Mustafa, T. "Ginger (Zingiber officinale) in rheumatism and musculoskeletal disorders." MEDICAL HYPOTHESES 1992 Dec;39(4):342-8.

90. Srivastava, K.C., Mustafa, T. "Ginger (Zingiber officinale) and rheumatic disorders." MEDICAL HYPOTHESES 1989 May; 29(1):25-8.

91. Suekawa, M., Yuasa, K., Isono, M., Sone, H., Ikeya, Y., Sakakibara, I., Aburada, M., Hosoya, E. ["Pharmacological studies on ginger. IV. Effect of (6)-shogaol on the arachidonic cascade"] NIPPON YAKURIGAKU ZASSHI. FOLIA PHARMACOLOGICA JAPONICA 1986 Oct;88(4):263-9.

92. Srivastava, K.C. "Effect of onion and ginger consumption on platelet thromboxane pro- duction in humans." PROSTAGLANDINS LEUKOTRIENES AND ESSENTIAL FATTY ACIDS 1989 Mar;35(3):183-5.

93. Srivastava, K.C. "Effects of aqueous extracts of onion, garlic and ginger on platelet aggregation and metabolism of arachidonic acid in the blood vascular system: in vitro study." PROSTAGLANDINS, LEUKOTRIENES AND MEDICINE 1984 Feb;13(2):227-35.

94. Srivastava, K.C. "Aqueous extracts of onion, garlic and ginger inhibit platelet aggregation and alter arachidonic acid metabolism." BIOMEDICA BIOCHIMICA ACTA 1984;43(8-9):S335-46.

95. Srivastava, K.C. "Isolation and effects of some ginger components of platelet aggregation and eicosanoid biosynthesis." PROSTAGLANDINS, LEUKOTRIENES AND MEDICINE 1986 Dec;25(2-3):187-98.

96. Flynn, D., et al. "Inhibition of human neutrophil 5 lipoxygenase activity by gingerdione, shogaol, capsaicin and related pungent compounds." PROSTAGLANDINS, LEUKOTRIENES AND MEDICINE 24:195-198, 1986.

97. Vellini, M., Desideri, D., Milanese, A., Omini, C., Daffonchio, L., Hernandez, A., Brunelli, G. "Possible involvement of eicosanoids in the pharmacological action of bromelain." ARZNEIMITTEL-FORSCHUNG 1986;36(1):110-12.

98. Taussig, S.J., Batkin, S. "Bromelain, the enzyme complex of pineapple (Ananas comosus) and its clinical application. An

update." JOURNAL OF ETHNOPHARMACOLOGY 1988 Feb-Mar; 22(2):191-203.

99. Ito, C., Yamaguchi, K., Shibutani, Y., Suzuki, K., Yamazaki, Y., Komachi, H., Ohnishi, H., Fujimura, H. ["Anti-inflammatory actions of proteases, bromelain, trypsin and their mixed preparation" (author's transl)] NIPPON YAKURIGAKU ZASSHI. FOLIA PHARMACOLOGICA JAPONICA 1979 Apr 20;75(3):227-37.

100. Duke, J.A. *Handbook of Biologically Active Phytochemicals and Their Activities.* CRC Press, Boca Raton, Fla., 1992, p. 69.

101. Kiuchi, F., Iwakami, S., Shibuya, M., Hanaoka, F., Sankawa, U. "Inhibition of prostaglandin and leukotriene biosynthesis by gingerols and diarylheptanoids." CHEMICAL AND PHARMACEUTICAL BULLETIN (Tokyo) 1992 Feb;40(2):387-91.

102. Govindarajan, V.S. "Ginger-Chemistry, technology, and quality evaluation: part 2." CRITICAL REVIEWS IN FOOD SCIENCE AND NUTRITION 1982;17(3):189-258 (p. 230), *citing* Hirahara, F. "Antioxidative activity of various spices on oils and fats. Antioxidative activity towards oxidation on storage and heating." JPN J NUTR 32(1),1, 1974; Food Sci Technol Abstr. 7(3) T 126, 1975.

103. Saito, Y., Kimura, Y., Sakamoto, T. "The antioxidant effects of petroleum ether soluble and insoluble fractions from spices." EIYO TO SHOKURYO 29 : 505-510 (1976).

104. Huang, J., et al. "Studies on the antioxidative activities of spices grown in Taiwan." CHUNG-KUO NUNG YEH HUA HSUEH HUI CHIH 1981 19(3-4).

105. Lee, Chan Juan, et al. "Studies on the antioxidative activities of spices grown in Taiwan." CHEMICAL ABSTRACTS Vol. 97, No. 3, 1982.

106. Han, B., et al. "Chemical and Biochemical Studies on Antioxidant Components of Ginseng." ADVANCES IN CHINESE MEDICINAL MATERIALS RESEARCH (485-498) (1985).

107. Lee, Y.B., Kim, Y.S., Ashmor, C.R. "Antioxidant property in Ginger Rhizome and its application to meat products." JOURNAL OF FOOD SCIENCE 51(1):20-23 (1986).

108. Ibid., citing Kihara, Y., and Inoue, T., "Antioxidant activity of spice powders in foods," citing CHEMICAL ABSTRACTS 1961 (19) 59:13276.

109. Ibid., citing Fujio et al. "Prevention of lipid oxidation in freeze dried foods.111 Antioxidative effects of spices and vegetables." CHEMICAL ABSTRACTS (1971) 74:2846.

110. Govindarajan, V.S. "Ginger—Chemistry, technology, and quality evaluation: part 1." CRITICAL REVIEWS IN FOOD SCIENCE AND NUTRITION 1982;17(1):1-96, citing Sethi, S.C., Aggarwal, J.S. "Stabilization of edible fats by spices and condiments." J SCI IND RES Sect B 11, 468 1952.

111. Mene' P Simonson, M.S., Dunn, M.J. "Eicosanoids, mesangial contraction, and intracellular signal transduction." TOHOKU JOURNAL OF EXPERIMENTAL MEDICINE 1992 Jan;166(1):57-73.

112. Busse, W.W., Gaddy, J.N. "The role of leukotriene antagonists and inhibitors in the treatment of airway disease." AMERICAN REVIEW OF RESPIRATORY DISEASE* 1991 May;143(5 Pt 2):S103-7.

113. Rask-Madsen, J., Bukhave, K., Laursen, L.S., Lauritsen, K. "5-Lipoxygenase inhibitors for the treatment of inflammatory bowel disease." AGENTS AND ACTIONS 1992; Spec No:C37-46.

114. McMillan, R.M., Walker, E.R. "Designing therapeutically effective 5-lipoxygenase inhibitors." TRENDS IN PHARMACOLOGICAL SCIENCES 1992 Aug; 13(8):323-30.

115. Ylikorkala, O., Viinikka, L. "The role of prostaglandins in obstetrical disorders." BAILLIERES CLINICAL OBSTETRICS AND GYNAECOLOGY 1992 Dec;6(4):809-27.

116. Hudson, N., Hawthorne, A.B., Cole, A.T., Jones, P.D., Hawkey, C.J. "Mechanisms of gastric and duodenal damage and protection." HEPATO-GASTROENTEROLOGY 1992 Feb;39 Suppl 1:31-6.

117. Fiddler, G.I., Lumley, P. "Preliminary clinical studies with thromboxane synthase inhibitors and thromboxane receptor blockers. A review." CIRCULATION 1990 Jan;81(1 Suppl):I69-78; discussion I79-80.

118. Hoet, B., et al. "Pharmacological manipulation of the thromboxane pathway in blood platelets." BLOOD COAGULATION AND FIBRINOLYSIS 1990 Jun;1(2):225-33.

119. Gresele, P., et al. "Thromboxane synthase inhibitors, thromboxane receptor antagonists

and dual blockers in thrombotic disorders." TRENDS IN PHARMACOLOGICAL SCIENCES 1991 Apr;12(4):158-63.

120. Backon, J. "Ginger: Inhibition of thromboxane synthetase and stimulation of prostacyclin: relevance for medicine and psychiatry." MEDICAL HYPOTHESES 1986 Jul;20(3):271-8.

121. Wilson, D.E. "Role of prostaglandins in gastroduodenal mucosal protection." JOURNAL OF CLINICAL GASTRO-ENTEROLOGY 1991;13 Suppl 1:S65-71.

122. Kimmey, M.B. "NSAIDs, ulcers, and prostaglandins." JOURNAL OF RHEUMATOLOGY 1992 Nov;19 Suppl 36:68-73.

123. Dajani, E.Z., Wilson, D.E., Agrawal, N.M. "Prostaglandins: An overview of the worldwide clinical experience." JOURNAL OF THE ASSOCIATION FOR ACADEMIC MINORITY PHYSICIANS 1991;2(1):23, 27-35.

124. Janusz, A.G., Janusz, A.J. "Prostaglandins: Viable therapy in gastric ulceration." SOUTH DAKOTA JOURNAL OF MEDICINE 1993 Feb;46(2):45-7.

125. Cryer, B., Feldman, M. "Effects of nonsteroidal anti-inflammatory drugs on endogenous gastrointestinal prostaglandins and therapeutic strategies for prevention and treatment of nonsteroidal anti-inflammatory drug-induced damage." ARCHIVES OF INTERNAL MEDICINE 1992 Jun; 152(6):1145-55.

126. Brzozowski, T. ["Gastro-protection in vivo and in vitro."] PATOLOGIA POLSKA 1992;43(1):1-9.

127. Camu, F., Van Lersberghe, C., Lauwers, M.H. "Cardiovascular risks and benefits of perioperative nonsteroidal anti-inflammatory drug treatment." DRUGS 1992;44 Suppl 5:42-51.

128. Kharazi, A.I., Pishel', I.N. ["The role of arachidonic acid derivatives in the system of immunity and its changes in aging."] FIZIOLOGICHESKII ZHURNAL 1990 Jan-Feb;36(1):107-13.

129. Thomsen, M.K., Ahnfelt-Ronne, I. ["Leukotrienes. A review of the significance for disease in man and the possibilities for therapeutic intervention."] UGESKRIFT FOR LAEGER 1991 Jan 14;153(3):173-6.

130. Droge, W., Wolf, M., Hacker-Shahin, B., Kriegbaum, H., Benninghoff, B., Gmunder, H., Eck, H.P., Mihm, S. "Immunomodulatory action of eicosanoids and other small molecular weight products of macrophages." ANNALI DELL ISTITUTO SUPERIORE DI SANITA 1991;27(1):67-9.

131. Claesson, H.E., Odlander, B., Jakobsson, P.J. "Leukotriene B4 in the immune system." INTERNATIONAL JOURNAL OF IMMUNOPHARMACOLOGY 1992 Apr;14(3):441-9.

132. Janniger, C.K., Racis, S.P. "The arachidonic acid cascade: An immunologically based review." JOURNAL OF MEDICINE 1987;18(2):69-80.

133. Rola-Pleszczynski, M. ["Regulation of the immune response using leukotrienes."] UNION MEDICALE DU CANADA 1989 May-Jun;118(3):111-3.

134. Srivastava, K.C. "Effects of aqueous extracts of onion, garlic and ginger on platelet aggregation and metabolism of arachidonic acid in the blood vascular system: in vitro study." PROSTAGLANDINS, LEUKOTRIENES AND MEDICINE 1984 Feb;13(2):227-35 (p.230).

135. Piacentini, G.L., Kaliner, M.A. "The potential roles of leukotrienes in bronchial asthma." AMERICAN REVIEW OF RESPIRATORY DISEASE 1991 May;143(5 Pt 2):S96-9.

136. Musser, J.H., Kreft, A.F. "5-lipoxygenase: Properties, pharmacology, and the quinolinyl(bridged)aryl class of inhibitors." JOURNAL OF MEDICINAL CHEMISTRY 1992 Jul 10;35(14):2501-24.

137. Nattero, G., Allais, G., De Lorenzo, C., Benedetto, C., Zonca, M., Melzi, E., Massobrio, M. "Relevance of prostaglandins in true menstrual migraine." HEADACHE 1989 Apr;29(4):233-8.

138. Benedetto, C. "Eicosanoids in primary dysmenorrhea, endometriosis and menstrual migraine." GYNECOLOGICAL ENDOCRINOLOGY 1989;3(1):71-94.

139. Vardi, Y., Rabey, I.M., Streifler, M., Schwartz, A., Lindner, H.R., Zor, U. "Migraine attacks. Alleviation by an inhibitor of prostaglandin synthesis and action." NEUROLOGY 1976 May;26(5):447-50.

140. Parantainen, J., Vapaatalo, H., Hokkanen, E. "Relevance of prostaglandins in migraine." CEPHALALGIA 1985 May;5 Suppl 2:93-7.

141. LaMancusa, R., Pulcinelli, F.M., Ferroni, P., Lenti, L., Manzari, G., Pauri, F., Rizzo, P.A., Gazzaniga, P.P., Pontieri, G.M. "Blood leukotrienes in headache: Correlation with platelet activity." HEADACHE 1991 Jun;31(6):409-14.

142. Rabey, J.M., Vardi, Y., Van Dyck, D., Streifler, M. "Ophthalmoplegic migraine: Amelioration by Flufenamic acid, a prostaglandin inhibitor." OPHTHALMOLOGICA 1977;175(3):148-52.

143. Beasley, J.D., Swift, J. *The Kellogg Report. The Impact of Nutrition, Environment & Lifestyle of the Health of Americans.* Institute of Health Policy Bard College, Annandale on Hudson, New York, 1989, p. 7G:353.

144. Murray, M., Pizzorno, J. *Encyclopedia of Natural Medicine.* Pima Publishing, Rocklin, Calif., 1991, p. 447.

145. Ibid., p. 492.

146. *Townsend Letter for Doctors,* February/March 1993, citing *Family Practice News,* October 15,1992.

147. Public Citizen Health Research Group, April 1993, Vol. 9, No. 4.

148. Beasley, J.D., Swift, J. *The Kellogg Report. The Impact of Nutrition, Environment & Lifestyle of the Health of Americans.* Institute of Health Policy Bard College, Annandale on Hudson, New York, 1989, p. 7D:335.

149. Castleman, M. *An Aspirin A Day: What You Can Do to Prevent Heart Attack, Stroke, and Cancer,* Hyperion, New York, 1993, pp 4-5.

150. Suekawa, M., et al. "Platelet aggregation inhibiting drug containing [6]-shogaol." CHEMICAL ABSTRACTS 109(11) 1988.

151. *New York Times,* Sept, 22, 1992.

152. Jenkins, R.R. "Free Radical Chemistry Relationship to Exercise." SPORTS MEDICINE 5: 156-170 (1988).

153. Eldershaw, T.P., Colquhoun, E.Q., Dora, K.A. Peng, Z.C., Clark, M.G. "Pungent principles of ginger (Zingiber officinale) are thermogenic in the perfused rat hindlimb." INTERNATIONAL JOURNAL OF OBESITY 1992 Oct;16(10):755-63.

154. Huang, Q., Matsuda, H., Sakai, K., Yamahara, J., Tamai, Y. ["The effect of ginger on serotonin induced hypothermia and diarrhea."] YAKUGAKU ZASSHI. JOURNAL OF THE PHARMACEUTICAL SOCIETY OF JAPAN 1990 Dec;110(12):936-42.

155. Suekawa, M., Ishige, A., Yuasa, K., Sudo, K., Aburada, M., Hosoya, E. "Pharmacological studies on ginger. I. Pharmacological actions of pungent constitutents, (6)-gingerol and (6)-shogaol." JOURNAL OF PHARMACOBIO-DYNAMICS 1984 Nov;7(11):836-48.

155a. Onogi, T., Minami, M., Kuraishi, Y., Satoh, M. "Capsaicin-like effect of (6)-shogoal on substance P-containing primary afferents of rats: A possible mechanism of its analgesic action." NEUROPHARMACOLOGY 1992;31(11):1165-69.

156. Yamahara, J., Miki, K., Chisaka, T., Sawada, T., Fujimura, H., Tomimatsu, T., Nakano, K., Nohara, T. "Cholagogic effect of ginger and its active constituents." JOURNAL OF ETHNOPHARMACOLOGY 1985 May;13(2):217-25, citing Stary, Z., (1925) "Uber Erregung der Warmenerven durch Pharmaka." ARCHIV FUR EXPERIMENTELLE PHATHOLOGIE UND PHARMAKOLOGIE 105, 76-87.

157. Ibid., citing Jancsó-Gábor, A., and Szolcsányi, J. (1970) "Action of rare earth metals complexes on neurogenic as well as on bradykinin-induced inflammation." JOURNAL OF PHARMACY AND PHARMACOLOGY 22, 366-371.

158. Ibid., citing Jancsó-Gábor, A. (1980) "Anaesthesia like condition and or potentiation of hexobarbitol sleep produced by pungent agents in normal and capsaicin-desensitized rats." ACTA PHYSIOLOGICA ACADEMIAE SCIENTIARUM HUNGARICAE 55, 57-62.

159. Ibid., citing Szolcsányi, J., and Jancsó-Gábor, A. (1973) "Capsaicin and other pungent agents as pharamacological tools in studies on thermoregulation." In E. Schönbaum and P. Lomax (eds), *The Pharmacology Of Thermoregulation and Drug Action,* Karger, Basel, p. 395-409.

160. Shiba, M., et al. "Antiulcer furanogermenone extraction from ginger." CHEM ABSTRACTS Vol 106, No 6, 1987.

161. Yamahara, J., Hatakeyama, S., Taniguchi, K., Kawamura, M., Yoshikawa, M. ["Stomachic principles in ginger. II. Pungent and anti-ulcer effects of low polar constituents isolated from ginger, the dried rhizoma of Zingiber officinale Roscoe cultivated in Taiwan. The absolute stereostructure of a new

diarylheptanoid."] YAKUGAKU ZASSHI. JOURNAL OF THE PHARMACEUTICAL SOCIETY OF JAPAN 1992 Sep;112(9): 645-55).

162. Yamahara, J., Mochizuki, M., Rong, H.Q., Matsuda, H., Fujimura, H. "The anti-ulcer effect in rats of ginger constituents." JOURNAL OF ETHNOPHARMACOLOGY 1988 Jul-Aug;23(2-3):299-304.

163. Ibid., citing Ogiso, A., et al. (1978) "Isolation and structure of an anti-peptic ulcer diterpene from a Thai medicinal plant." CHEMICAL PHARMACEUTICAL BULLETIN 26, 3117-3123.

164. Al-Yahya, M.A., Rafatullah, S., Mossa, J.S., Ageel, A.M., Parmar, N.S., Tariq, M. "Gastroprotective activity of ginger, zingiber officinale rosc., in albino rats." AMERICAN JOURNAL OF CHINESE MEDICINE 1989;17(1-2):51-6.

165. Ibid., citing Enchi et al. "Novel diterpenelactones with anti-peptic ulcer activity from Croton sublyratus." CHEMICAL PHARMACEUTICAL BULLETIN 28(1), 227-234, 1980.

166. Ibid., citing Trease, E., and Evans, W. *Pharmacognosy* (11th ed.) Baillare Tindall, London, 1978, p. 632-37.

167. Wu, H., Ye, D., Bai, Y., Zhao, Y. ["Effect of dry ginger and roasted ginger on experimental gastric ulcers in rats."] CHUNG-KUO CHUNG YAO TSA CHIH [CHINA JOURNAL OF CHINESE MATERIA] 1990 May;15(5):278-80, 317-8.

168. Backon, J. "Ginger and carbon dioxide as thromboxane synthetase inhibitors:potential utility in treating peptic ulceration." GUT (1987) 28:1323.

169. Sakai, K., et al. "Effect of extracts of Zingiberaceae herbs on gastric secretion in rabbits." CHEM. PHARM. BULL 37(1) 215-217 (1989).

170. Sertie, J., Basile, A., et al. "Preventive anti-ulcer activity of the rhizome extract of Zingiber officinale." FITOTHERAPIA 1992 63:1 55-59.

171. Ibid., citing Gilbert V.A., et al., HORMONE AND METABOLIC RES 15, 320 (1983).

171a. Yoshikawa, M., Hatakeyama, S., Taniguchi, K., Matuda, H., Yamahara, J. "6-Gingesulfonic acid, a new anti-ulcer principle, and gingerglycolipids A,B and C, three new monoacyldigalactosylglycerols from Zingiberis rhizoma originating in Taiwan." CHEMICAL & PHARMACEUTICAL BULLETIN 1992;40(8):2239-41.

172. Sertie, J., Basile, A., et al. "Preventive anti-ulcer activity of the rhizome extract of Zingiber officinale." FITOTHERAPIA 1992 63:155-59, citing Bennett T., INT J TISSUE REACTION 5,237 (1983).

173. Bright-Asare, P., Habte, T., Yirgou, B., Benjamin, J. "Prostaglandins, H2-receptor antagonists and peptic ulcer disease." DRUGS 1988;35 Suppl 3:1-9.

174. Stec, L.F. "Peptic Ulcer-The Price of Stress." *Bestways* April 1980 p. 38-40.

175. "The 100 drugs by U.S. sales." *Medical Advertising News*, May 1993.

176. Koop, H., Eissele, R. ["Reduction of gastric acid secretion: pathophysiologic and clinically relevant sequelae."] ZEITSCHRIFT FUR GASTROENTEROLOGIE 1991 Nov;29(11):613-7.

176a. Chaturvedi, G.N., Mahadeo, P., Agrawal, A.K., Gupta, J.P. "Some clinical and experimental studies on whole root of glycyrrhiza glabra linn. (yashtimadhu) in peptic ulcer." INDIAN MED GAZ 113 : 200-205 (1979).

176b. Rees, W.D., Rhodes, J., Wright, J.E., Stamford, L.F., Bennett, A. "Effect of deglycyrrhizinated liquorice on gastric mucosal damage by aspirin." SCANDINAVIAN JOURNAL OF GASTROENTEROLOGY 1979;14(5):605-7.

176c. Das, S.K., Das, V., Gulati, A.K., Singh, V.P. "Deglycyrrhizinated liquorice in aphthous ulcers." JOURNAL OF THE ASSOCIATION OF PHYSICIANS OF INDIA 1989 Oct; 37(10):647.

176d. Morgan, A.G., McAdam, W.A., Pacsoo, C., Darnborough, A. "Comparison between cimetidine and Caved-S in the treatment of gastric ulceration, and subsequent maintenance therapy." GUT 1982 Jun;23 (6):545-51.

176e. Glick, L. "Deglycyrrhizinated liquorice for peptic ulcer." [letter] LANCET 1982 Oct 9;2(8302):817.

177. *Borderlines in Medical Science. Inroductory lecture delivered before the medical class of Medical School of Harvard U.* 6. Nov 1861, in Medical Essays, p. 255 (pg.

297) citing Green Pharmacy.

178. Yamahara, J., Huang, Q.R., Li, Y.H., Xu, L., Fujimura, H. "Gastrointestinal motility enhancing effect of ginger and its active constituents." CHEMICAL AND PHARMACEUTICAL BULLETIN 1990 Feb;38(2):430-1.

179. Ibid., citing Yamahara, J. et al. PHYTOTHERAPY RESEARCH 3, 70 (1989).

180. Nes, I.F., Skjekvale, R., et al. "The effect of natural spices and oleoresins on Lactobacillus plantarum and Staphylococcus aureus." MICROBIAL ASSOCIATIONS AND INTERACTIONS IN FOOD 435-440.

181. Hikino, H., Kiso, Y., Kato, N., Hamada, Y., Shioiri, T., Aiyama, R., Itokawa, H., Kiuchi, F., Sankawa, U. "Antihepatotoxic actions of gingerols and diarylheptanoids." J ETHNOPHARMACOL 1985 Sep;14(1):31-9.

182. Yamahara, J., Rong, H.Q., Naitoh, Y., Kitani, T., Fujimura, H. "Inhibition of cytotoxic drug-induced vomiting in suncus by a ginger constituent." J ETHNO-PHARMACOL 1989 Dec;27(3):353-5.

183. Pace, J.C. "Oral ingestion of encapsulated ginger and reported self-care actions for the relief of chemotherapy-associated nausea and vomiting." DISS ABSTR INT (SCI) 1987; 47(8):3297.

184. Liu, W.H. "Ginger root, a new antiemetic." (letter; comment) ANAESTHESIA 1990 Dec;45(12):1085.

185. Backon, J. "Ginger as an antiemetic: Possible side effects due to its thromboxane synthetase activity." [letter] ANAESTHESIA 1991 Aug;46(8):705-6.

186. Grontved, A., Brask, T., Kambskard, J., Hentzer, E. "Ginger root against seasickness. A controlled trial on the open sea." ACTA OTO-LARYNGOLOGICA 1988 Jan-Feb; 105(1-2):45-9.

187. Mowrey, D.B., Clayson, D.E. "Motion sickness, ginger, and psychophysics." LANCET 1982 Mar 20;1(8273):655-7.

188. Grontved, A., Hentzer, E. "Vertigo-reducing effect of ginger root. A controlled clinical study." ORL; JOURNAL OF OTO-RHINO-LARYNGOLOGY AND ITS RELATED SPECIALTIES 1986;48(5):282-6.

189. Backon, J. "Ginger in preventing nausea and vomiting of pregnancy; a caveat due to its thromboxane synthetase activity and effect on testosterone binding." [letter;] EUROPEAN JOURNAL OF OBSTETRICS, GYNECOLOGY, AND REPRODUCTIVE BIOLOGY 1991 Nov 26;42(2):163-4.

190. Bone, M.E., Wilkinson, D.J., Young, J.R., McNeil, J., Charlton S. "Ginger root-A new antiemetic. The effect of ginger root on postoperative nausea and vomiting after major gynaecological surgery." ANAESTHESIA 1990 Aug;45(8):669-71.

190a. Phillips, S., Ruggier, R., Hutchinson, S.E. "Zingiber officinale (Ginger)—An antiemetic for day case surgery." ANAESTHESIA 1993;48(8):715-17.

191. Fischer-Rasmussen, W., Kjaer, S.K., Dahl, C. Asping, U. "Ginger treatment of hyperemesis gravidarum." EUROPEAN JOURNAL OF OBSTETRICS, GYNECOLOGY, AND REPRODUCTIVE BIOLOGY 1991 Jan 4;38(1):19-24.

192. *Physicians Desk Reference* (47th ed), Medical Economics, 1993, p. 1097.

193. Ibid., p. 2323.

194. Brooks, W.S. "Short- and long-term management of peptic ulcer disease: Current role of H2-antagonists." HEPATO GASTRO-ENTEROLOGY 1992 Feb;39 Suppl 1:47-52.

195. Wood, C.D., Manno, J.E., et al. "Comparison of efficacy of Ginger with various antimotion sickness drugs." CLINICAL RESEARCH PRACTICES & DRUG REGUATORY AFFAIRS 6(2), 129-36 (1988).

196. Stewart, J.J., Wood, M.J., Wood, C.D., Mims, M.E. "Effects of ginger on motion sickness susceptibility and gastric function." PHARMACOLOGY 1991;42(2):111-20.

196a. Phillips, S., Hutchinson, S., Ruggier, R. "Zingiber officinale does not affect gastric emptying rate: A randomised, placebo-controlled, crossover trial." ANAESTHESIA 1993;48(5):393-95.

197. *Physicians Desk Reference* (47th ed), Medical Economics, 1993, p. 1952.

198. Huang, Q.R., Iwamoto, M., Aoki, S., Tanaka, N., Tajima, K., Yamahara, J., Takaishi, Y., Yoshida, M., Tomimatsu, T., Tamai, Y. "Anti-5-hydroxytryptamine effect of galanolactone, diterpenoid isolated from ginger." CHEMICAL AND PHARMACEUTICAL BULLETIN (Tokyo) 1991 Feb;39(2):397-9.

199. Koltai, M., Mecs, I., Kasa, M. "On the anti-inflammatory effect of sendai virus inoculation." ARCHIVES OF VIROLOGY

1981;67(1):91-5.

200. Karevina, T.G., Khokholia, V.P., Shevchuk, I.M. ["Effects of serotonin and stress on the state of the gastric mucosa in rats with the intact and transsected vagus nerve."] BIULLETEN EKSPERIMENTALNOI BIOLOGII I MEDITSINY 1989 Nov; 108(11):545-7.

201. Spannhake, E.W., Levin, J.L., Mellion, B.T., Gruetter, C.A., Hyman, A.L., Kadowitz, P.J. "Reversal of 5HT-induced broncho-constriction by PGI2: Distribution of central and peripheral actions." JOURNAL OF APPLIED PHYSIOLOGY: RESPIRATORY, ENVIRONMENTAL 1980 Sep;49(3):521-7.

202. Lichtenthal, P.R., Wade, L.D., Rossi, E.C. "The effect of ketanserin on blood pressure and platelets during cardiopulmonary bypass." ANESTHESIA AND ANALGESIA 1987 Nov;66(11):1151-4.

203. Heistad, D.D., Harrison, D.G., Armstrong, M.L. "Serotonin and experimental vascular disease." INTERNATIONAL JOURNAL OF CARDIOLOGY 987 Feb;14(2):205-12.

204. Schror, K. Braun, M. "Platelets as a source of vasoactive mediators." STROKE 1990 Dec;21(12 Suppl):IV32-5.

205. Christopher, J. School of Natural Healing. Bi-World, Provo, Utah, 1976.

206. Motono, M. "Manufacture of topical cosmetics and pharmaceuticals containing ginger extracts as absorption accelerators." CHEMICAL ABSTRACTS Vol 112, 223137 1990.

207. Srivastava, K.C., Mustafa, T. "Ginger (Zingiber officinale) in rheumatism and musculoskeletal disorders." MEDICAL HYPOTHESES 1992 Dec;39(4):342-8, citing Dorso C et al., "Chinese Food and platelets." NEW ENGLAND JOURNAL OF MEDICINE 303:756-757, 1980.

208. Brody, Jane, *New York Times,* April 1, 1993.

209. Dalton, H.P., Nottebart, H.C., Jr., INTERPRETATIVE MEDICAL MICROBIOLOGY, 1986;501.

210. Feroz, H. et al. "Review of scientific studies of anthelmintics from plants." JOURNAL OF SCI. RES. PL & MED. 3:1 1982, 6-12.

211. Tietze, P.E., Tietze, P.H. "The round-worm, Ascaris lumbricoides." PRIMARY CARE; CLINICS IN OFFICE PRACTICE 1991 Mar;18(1):25-41.

212. Markell, E.K., Voge, M., John, D.T. *Medical Parasitology* (6th ed), W.B. Saunders Co., Philadelphia, 1986, p. 165.

213. Ibid., p. 166.

214. Raj, R. "Screening of some indigenous plants for anthelmintic action against human ascaris lumbricoides." INDIAN JOURNAL PHYSIOLOGY AND PHARMACOLOGY 18(2): 129-131, 1974.

215. Markell, E., Voge, M., John, D. *Medical Parasitology,* W.B. Saunders Co., Philadelphia, 1986, p. 243.

216. Ibid., p. 167.

217. Capron, A.R. "Immunity to schistosomes." CURRENT OPINION IN IMMUNOLOGY 1992 Aug;4(4):419-24.

218. Markell, E., Voge, M., John, D. *Medical Parasitology,* W.B. Saunders Co., Philadelphia, 1986, p. 167.

219. Dean, M., Dhaliwal, A., Jones, W. "Effects of Zingiberacae rhizome extract on the infectivity of cyanophage LPP-1." TRANS- ACTIONS OF THE ILLINOIS STATE ACADEMY OF SCIENCE 80:April 10-12, 1987.

220. Endo, K., et al. "Structures of antifungal diarylheptenones, gingerenones A,B, C and isogingerenone B, isolated from the rhizomes of Zingiber officinale." PHYTOCHEMISTRY 1990, Vol. 29, No. 3, pp. 797-799.

221. Govindarajan, V.S. "Ginger-Chemistry, technology, and quality evaluation: part 2." CRITICAL REVIEWS IN FOOD SCIENCE AND NUTRITION 1982;17(3):189-258 (p. 230), citing Hitokoto, H., et al. "Inhibitory effects of spices on growth and toxin production of toxigenic fungi." APP ENVIRON MICROBIOL 39(4), 818, 1980.

222. Guérin, J.C., Réveillère, H.P. "Activité antifongique d'extraits végétaux à usage thérapeutique 1. Etude de 41 extraits sur 9 souches fongiques." ANN PHARMACEUTIQUES FRANÇAISES 1984, 42, no. 6, pp. 553-9.

223. CHEMICAL ABSTRACTS: "Antihistaminic substance from ginger." TOYODA ISAO (Japan) 69 08,561 21 Apr 1969.

223a. Ames, B. "Dietary Carcinogens and Anticarcinogens." SCIENCE 1983 Sept. 23; Vol 221 1256-1264.

224. Morita, S., et al. (1978) "Studies on natural desmutagens: Screening for vegetable and fruit factors active in activation of mutagenic pyrolysis products from amino acids." AGRIC BIOL CHEM 42 (6), 1235-1238.

225. Nakamura, H., Yamamoto, T. "Mutagen and anti-mutagen in ginger, Zingiber officinale." MUTATION RESEARCH 1982 Feb;103(2):119-26.

226. Sakai, Y., et al. "Effects of medicinal plant extracts from Chinese herbal medicines on the mutagenic activity of benzo(a)pyrene." MUTATION RESEARCH 206 (1988) 327-334.

227. Kada, T., Morita, M., Inoue, T. (1978) "Antimutagenic action of vegetable factor(s) on the mutagenic principle of tryptophan pyrolysate" MUTATION RESEARCH 53, 351-353.

228. Yamaguchi, T. "Desmutagenic activity of peroxidase on autoxidized linolenic acid." AGRIC BIOL CHEM 44(4), 959-961, 1980.

229. Nagabhushan, M., Amonkar, A.J., Bhide, S.V. "Mutagenicity of gingerol and shogaol and antimutagenicity of zingerone in Salmonella/microsome assay." CANCER LETTERS 1987 Aug;36(2):221-33.

230. Ohta, S., et al. "Studies on Chemical Protectors Against Radiation. XXV. Radioprotective Activities of Various Crude Drugs." YAKUGAKU ZASSHI 107(1) 70-75 (1987).

231. Unnikrihnan, M. "Tumour reducing and anticarcinogenic activity of selected spices." CANCER LETTERS, 51 (1990) 85-89.

232. Ibid., citing Unnikrihnan, M., Kuttan, R. (1988) "Cytotoxicity of extracts of spices to cultured cells." NUTR CANCER 11 (4), 251.

233. Ibid., citing Goodpasture, C., Arrighi, F. (1976) "Effects of food seasoning on the cycle and chromosomemorphology of mamalian cells in vitro with special reference to turmeric." FOOD COSMET TOXICOL14, 2.

233a. Castleman, M. *An Aspirin A Day: What You Can Do to Prevent Heart Attack, Stroke, and Cancer*, Hyperion, New York, 1993, p. 79.

234. Yamazaki, M., Nishimura, T. "Induction of Neutrophil Accumulation by Vegetable Juice." BIOSCI. BIOTECH. BIOCHEM (1), 150-151, 1992.

235. Govindarajan, V.S. "Ginger-Chemistry, technology, and quality evaluation: part 2." CRITICAL REVIEWS IN FOOD SCIENCE AND NUTRITION 1982;17(3):189-258 (p. 230), citing Gujral, S., et al. "Effect of ginger (Zingiber officinale Roscoe) oleoresin on serum and hepatic cholesterol levels in cholesterol- fed rats." NUTR REP INT 17(2), 183, 1978.

236. Tanabe, M., Chen, Y.D., Saito, K., Kano, Y. "Cholesterol biosynthesis inhibitory component from Zingiber officinale Roscoe." CHEMICAL AND PHARMACEUTICAL BULLETIN (Tokyo) 1993 Apr;41(4):710-3.

237. Giri, J., et al. MED & AROMAT PLANTS ABSTRACTS Vol. 7, No. 5, 1985.

238. Ally, M. "The pharmacological action of Zingiber officinale." CHEMICAL ABSTRACTS 61(1964) 6047.

239. Kobayashi, M., Ishida, Y., Shoji, N., Ohizumi, Y. "Cardiotonic action of [8]-gingerol, an activator of the Ca++-pumping adenosine triphosphatase of sarcoplasmic reticulum, in guinea pig atrial muscle." JOURNAL OF PHARMACOLOGY AND EXPERIMENTAL THERAPEUTICS 1988 Aug;246(2):667-73.

240. Kobayashi, M., Shoji, N., Ohizumi, Y. "Gingerol, a novel cardiotonic agent, activates the Ca2+-pumping ATPase in skeletal and cardiac sarcoplasmic reticulum." BIO-CHIMICA ET BIOPHYSICA ACTA 1987 Sep 18;903(1):96-102.

241. Shoji, N., Iwasa, A., Takemoto, T., Ishida, Y., Ohizumi, Y. "Cardiotonic principles of ginger (Zingiber officinale Roscoe)." JOURNAL OF PHARMACEUTICAL SCIENCES 1982 Oct;71(10):1174-5.

242. Yamahara, J., Miki, K., Chisaka, T., Sawada, T., Fujimura, H., Tomimatsu, T., Nakano, K., Nohara, T. "Cholagogic effect of ginger and its active constituents." JOURNAL OF ETHNOPHARMACOLOGY 1985 May;13(2):217-25, citing Kasahara, Y., et al. (1983) "Pharmacological actions of Pinellia Tubers and Zingiber rhizomes." SHOYAKUGAKU ZASSHI 37, 73-83.

243. Backon, J. "Possible utility of a thromboxane synthetase inhibitor in preventing penile vascular changes and impotence during aging." ARCHIVES OF ANDROLOGY 1988; 20:101-2.

244. Backon, J. "Mechanism of analgesic effect of clonidine in the treatment of dysmenor-rhea." MEDICAL HYPOTHESES 1991 Nov;36(3):223-4.

245. Xiong, H.X. ["Changes in multihormones in treating male sterility with acupuncture and indirect moxibustion using ginger slices on the skin."] CHUNG HSI I CHIEH HO TSA CHIH 1986 Dec;6(12):726-7, 708.

246. Cai, R., Zhou, A., Gao, H. ["Study on correction of abnormal fetal position by applying ginger paste at zhihying acupoint A. Report of 133 cases."] CHEN TZU YEN CHIU [ACUPUNCTURE RESEARCH] 1990;15(2):89-91.

247. Personal communication with Julie Plunkett.

248. Govindarajan, V.S. "Ginger—Chemistry, technology, and quality evaluation: part 1." CRITICAL REVIEWS IN FOOD SCIENCE AND NUTRITION 1982;17(1):1-96 (p. 4).

249. Ibid., p. 21, citing Scott, P., Kennedy, R. "Analysis of spices and herbs for aflatoxins." CAN INST FOOD SCI TECHNOL J. 8(2), 124, 1975.

250. Ibid., p. 23.

251. Ibid., p. 26.

252. Ibid., p. 28.

253. Ye, D.J., Ding, A.W., Guo, R. ["A research on the constituents of ginger in various preparations."] CHUNG-KUO CHUNG YAO TSA CHIH [CHINA JOURNAL OF CHINESE MATERIA] 1989 May;14(5): 278-80, 318.

254. Govindarajan, V.S. "Ginger-Chemistry, technology, and quality evaluation: part 2." CRITICAL REVIEWS IN FOOD SCIENCE AND NUTRITION 1982;17(3):189-258 (p. 227).

255. Govindarajan, V.S. "Ginger-Chemistry, technology, and quality evaluation: part 2." CRITICAL REVIEWS IN FOOD SCIENCE AND NUTRITION 1982;17(3):189-258 (p. 221).

256. Allen, K.L., Molan, P.C., Reid, G.M. "A survey of the antibacterial activity of some New Zealand honeys." JOURNAL OF PHARMACY AND PHARMACOLOGY 1991 Dec;43(12):817-22.

257. Jeddar, A., Kharsany, A., Ramsaroop, U.G., Bhamjee, A., Haffejee, I.E., Moosa, A. "The antibacterial action of honey. An in vitro study." SOUTH AFRICAN MEDICAL JOURNAL 1985 Feb 16;67(7):257-8.

258. Willix, D.J., Molan, P.C., Harfoot, C.G. "A comparison of the sensitivity of wound-infecting species of bacteria to the anti-bacterial activity of manuka honey and other honey." JOURNAL OF APPLIED BACTERIOLOGY 1992 Nov;73(5):388-94.

259. Gribel', N.V., Pashinskii, V.G. ["The antitumor properties of honey."] VOPROSY ONKOLOGII 1990;36(6):704-9.

260. Wellford, T.E., Eadie, T., Llewellyn, G.C. "Evaluating the inhibitory action of honey on fungal growth, sporulation, and aflatoxin production." ZEITSCHRIFT FUR LEBENSMITTEL-UNTERSUCHUNG UND-FORSCHUNG 1978 Jun 28; 166(5):280-3.

261. Obaseiki-Ebor, E.E., Afonya, T.C. "In-vitro evaluation of the anticandidiasis activity of honey distillate (HY-1) compared with that of some antimycotic agents." JOURNAL OF PHARMACY AND PHARMACOLOGY 1984 Apr;36(4):283-4.

262. Efem, S.E., Udoh, K.T., Iwara, C.I. "The antimicrobial spectrum of honey and its clinical significance." INFECTION 1992 Jul-Aug;20(4):227-9.

263. Ndayisaba, G., Bazira, L., Habonimana, E. ["Treatment of wounds with honey. 40 cases."] PRESSE MEDICALE 1992 Oct 3;21(32): 1516-8.

264. Efem, S.E. "Clinical observations on the wound healing properties of honey." BRITISH JOURNAL OF SURGERY 1988 Jul;75(7):679-81.

265. Subrahmanyam, M. "Topical application of honey in treatment of burns." BRITISH JOURNAL OF SURGERY 1991 Apr;78(4):497-8.

266. Bergman, A., Yanai, J., Weiss, J., Bell, D., David, M.P. "Acceleration of wound healing by topical application of honey. An animal model." AMERICAN JOURNAL OF SURGERY 1983 Mar;145(3):374-6.

267. Efem, S.E. "Recent advances in the management of Fournier's gangrene: Preliminary observations." [see comments] SURGERY 1993 Feb;113(2):200-4.

268. Phuapradit, W., Saropala, N. "Topical application of honey in treatment of abdominal wound disruption." AUSTRALIAN AND NEW ZEALAND JOURNAL OF OBSTETRICS AND GYNAECOLOGY 1992 Nov;32(4):381-4.

269. Ali, A.T., Chowdhury, M.N., Al Humayyd, M.S. "Inhibitory effect of natural

honey on Helicobacter pylori." TROPICAL GASTROENTEROLOGY 1991 Jul-Sep; 12(3):139-43.

270. Ali, A.T. "Prevention of ethanol-induced gastric lesions in rats by natural honey, and its possible mechanism of action." SCANDINAVIAN JOURNAL OF GASTROENTEROLOGY 1991 Mar;26(3):281-8.

271. Haffejee, I.E., Moosa, A. "Honey in the treatment of infantile gastroenteritis." BRITISH MEDICAL JOURNAL [CLINICAL RESEARCH ED.] 1985 Jun 22;290(6485):1866-7.

272. Samanta, A., Burden, A.C., Jones, G.R. "Plasma glucose responses to glucose, sucrose, and honey in patients with diabetes mellitus: An analysis of glycaemic and peak incremental indices." DIABETIC MEDICINE 1985 Sep;2(5):371-3.

273. Bornet, F., Haardt, M.J., Costagliola, D., Blayo, A., Slama, G. "Sucrose or honey at breakfast have no additional acute hyperglycaemic effect over an isoglucidic amount of bread in type 2 diabetic patients." DIABETOLOGIA 1985 Apr;28(4):213-7.

274. Shambaugh, P., Worthington, V., Herbert, J.H. "Differential effects of honey, sucrose, and fructose on blood sugar levels." [see comments] JOURNAL OF MANIPULATIVE AND PHYSIOLOGICAL THERAPEUTICS 1990 Jul-Aug;13(6):322-5.

275. Akhtar, M.S., Khan, M.S. "Glycaemic responses to three different honeys given to normal and alloxan-diabetic rabbits." JPMA. JOURNAL OF THE PAKISTAN MEDICAL ASSOCIATION 1989 Apr;39(4):107-13.

276. Obaseiki-Ebor, E.E., Afonya, T.C. "In-vitro evaluation of the anticandidiasis activity of honey distillate (HY-1) compared with that of some antimycotic agents." JOURNAL OF PHARMACY AND PHARMACOLOGY 1984 Apr;36(4):283-4.

277. *Science News*, Biomedicine section, Sept. 25, 1993, vol. 144.

278. Heinerman, J., *Heinerman's Encyclopedia of Fruits, Vegetables and Herbs*, Parker Publishing Co., West Nyack, N.Y.,1988, p. 154.

279. Govindarajan, V.S. "Ginger—Chemistry, technology, and quality evaluation: part 1." CRITICAL REVIEWS IN FOOD SCIENCE AND NUTRITION 1982;17(1):1-96 (p. 53), citing Winterton, D., Richardson, K. "An investigation into the chemical constituents of Queensland grown ginger." QUEENSL J AGRIC SCI 22, 205, 1965.

280. Heinerman, J., *The Complete Book of Spices*, Keats Publishing Inc., New Canaan, Conn, 1983, pp. 38-39.

281. *FDA Task Force Report*, Washington, D.C., June 15, 1993.

282. Carter, J.A. *Racketeering in Medicine: The Suppression of Alternatives.* Hampton Roads, 1992.

283. Cynthia Cotts, *The Nation*, Aug. 31/Sept. 7, 1992.

284. *New York Times*, Sept. 22, 1992.

285. *Natural Health*, January/February, p. 88.

286. "Earthsave Statistics From How To Win An Argument With A Meat Eater."

287. National Research Council, 1982. "Diet, Nutrition, and Cancer." National Academy Press, Washington, D.C., p. 55.

288. Kaiser Permanente Health Group, *Longevity*, June 1993.

289. Associated Press, *New York Times*, May 26, 1993.

290. Murray, M., 1991 SWHO Convention on Botanical Medicine.

291. Classen, D.C., et al. JAMA 11/27/91 Vol. 266, No. 20.

292. 1990 GAO (General Accounting Office) report, Washington, D.C.

293. Associated Press release, Dec. 22, 1992.

294. Little Rock Economic Conference, Associated Press release, Dec. 15, 1992.

295. *New York Times*, Sept. 22, 1992.

296. Brody, J. "Vitamin E Greatly Reduces Risk Of Heart Disease, Studies Suggest Best Results Found in Those Taking Large Doses." *New York Times*, May 20, 1993.

297. Toda, S., Kimura, M., et al. "Natural Antioxidants Antioxidative Components Isolated from Schizandra Fruit." SHOYAKUGAKU ZASSHI 42(2) 156-159 (1988).

298. Shalini, V.K., Srinivas, L. "Lipid Peroxide Induced DNA Damage: Protection by Turmeric (Curcuma longa)." MOLLECULAR AND CELLULAR BIOCHEMISTRY 77: 3-10 (1987).

299. Walker, M. "Pycnogenol: Powerful Antioxidant." *Natural Health*, July/August

1993, pp. 40-41.

300. Plyasunova, O.A., Pokrovsky, A.G., Rusakov, I.A., Baltina, L.A., Murinov, Y.I., Tolstikov, G.A. "Inhibition of HIV reproduction in cell cultures by glycyrrhizic acid." INTERNATIONAL CONFERENCE ON AIDS 1992 Jul 19-24;8(3):31.

301. Pliasunova, O.A., Egoricheva, I.N., Fediuk, N.V., Pokrovskii, A.G., Baltina, L.A., Murinov, Iu.I., Tolstikov, G.A. ["The anti-HIV activity of beta-glycyrrhizic acid."] "Izuchenie anti-VICh-aktivnosti beta-glitsirrizinovoi kisloty." VOPROSY VIRUSOLOGII 1992 Sep-Dec;37(5-6):235-8.

302. Shashikanth, K.N., Basappa, S.C., Sreenivasa Murthy, V. "A comparative study of raw garlic extract and tetracycline on caecal microflora and serum proteins of albino rats." FOLIA MICROBIOLOGICA (Praha) 1984;29(4):348-52.

303. Russin, W.A., Hoesly, J.D., Elson, C.E., Tanner, M.A., Gould, M.N. "Inhibition of rat mammary carcinogenesis by monoterpenoids." CARCINOGENESIS 1989 Nov;10(11):2161-4.

304. Elegbede, J.A., Elson, C.E., Qureshi, A., Tanner, M.A., Gould, M.N. "Inhibition of DMBA-induced mammary cancer by the monoterpene d-limonene." CARCINOGENESIS 1984 May;5(5):661-4.

305. *Larry King Live* (television show), aired 1992.

306. McCaleb, R. "Rational Regulation of Herbal Products Testimony Before The Subcommittee On Govenment Regulations." citing Snider, S. "Beware the unknown brew; herbal teas and toxicity." FDA CONSUMER, 1991 25(4):30-33.

307. McCaleb, R. "Rational Regulation of Herbal Products Testimony Before The Subcommittee On Govenment Regulations," citing *Innovations in Medicine #17,* Pharmaceutical Manufacturers Association.

308. Annual Meeting Federation of American Societies for Experimental Biology New Orleans, Louisiana, March 31, 1993 (two other high officials confirmed).

309. 1990 GAO (General Accounting Office) report, Washington, D.C.

310. "Medical Controversy," *Time* magazine, March 18, 1991.

311. Associated Press release, Chicago, May 12, 1993.

311a. Philip Holzberer, in editorial to the *New York Times,* January 7, 1993.

312. *Vegetarian Times*, February 1993.

313. Associated Press release, *NewYork Times,* Jaunary 2, 1993, page 1.

314. Duke, J.A. *Phytochemical Constituents of GRAS Herbs and Other Economic Plants* (Database), CRC Press, 1992.

315. Duke, J.A. *Handbook of Biologically Active Phytochemicals and Their Activities,* CRC Press, 1992, 183 pp.

Index

A

B

C

D

E

R

S

T

U

V

W

Z

About the Author

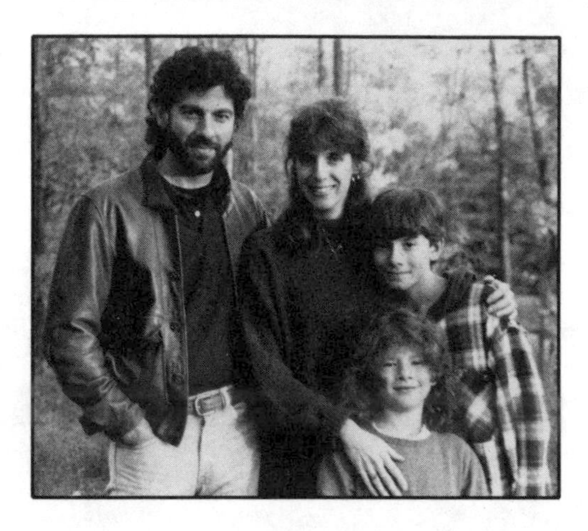

Paul Schulick is nationally recognized for the herbal research he calls "data base herbalism." Drawing from medical computer data bases such as Medline and Napralert, Paul supports his herbal theories and traditionally inspired formulations with international scientific data. His research ranges from the therapeutic value of sea herbs to discovering the healing powers of herbs commonly found in the spice cabinet. Paul has lectured throughout the United States on the impact of herbs and natural foods on our national health. He is a dedicated defender of alternative medicine and "freedom of choice" in health care.

Paul lives and works with his wife Barbi and their children Geremy and Rosalie in Brattleboro, Vermont.